MEDICAL
INTELLIGENCE
UNIT

MYOCARDIAL INJURY: LABORATORY DIAGNOSIS

Johannes Mair, M.D.
Bernd Puschendorf, M.D.
University of Innsbruck
Innsbruck, Austria

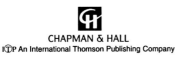

CHAPMAN & HALL
I(T)P An International Thomson Publishing Company

New York • Albany • Bonn • Boston • Cincinnati • Detroit • London • Madrid • Melbourne •
Mexico City • Pacific Grove • Paris • San Francisco • Singapore • Tokyo • Toronto • Washington

R.G. LANDES COMPANY
AUSTIN

MEDICAL INTELLIGENCE UNIT
MYOCARDIAL INJURY: LABORATORY DIAGNOSIS

R.G. LANDES COMPANY
Austin, Texas, U.S.A.

U.S. and Canada Copyright © 1997 R.G. Landes Company and Chapman & Hall

Please address all inquiries to the Publishers:
R.G. Landes Company, 909 Pine Street, Georgetown, Texas, U.S.A. 78626
Phone: 512/ 863 7762; FAX: 512/ 863 0081

North American distributor:
Chapman & Hall, 115 Fifth Avenue, New York, New York, U.S.A. 10003

CHAPMAN & HALL

U.S. and Canada ISBN: 0-412-11391-0

Library of Congress Cataloging-in-Publication Data
Mair, Johannes, 1962-
    Myocardial injury: laboratory diagnosis / Johannes Mair, Bernd Puschendorf.
        p. cm. — (Medical intelligence unit)
    Includes bibliographical references and index.
    ISBN 1-57059-303-5 (RGL-alk. paper); ISBN 0-412-11391-0 (CH-alk. paper)
    1. Myocardial infarction—Molecular diagnosis. 2. Diagnosis, Laboratory. I. Puschendorf, Bernd, 1942- . II. Title. III. Series.
        [DNLM: 1.Myocardial infarction—diagnosis. 2. Myocardial Infarction—physiopathology. 3. Biological Markers. 4. Diagnosis, Laboratory. WG 300 M228L 1996]
RC685.I6M266 1996
616.1'237'075—dc20
DNLM/DLC   96-27642
for Library of Congress   CIP

Publisher's Note

R.G. Landes Company publishes six book series: *Medical Intelligence Unit, Molecular Biology Intelligence Unit, Neuroscience Intelligence Unit, Tissue Engineering Intelligence Unit, Biotechnology Intelligence Unit* and *Environmental Intelligence Unit.* The authors of our books are acknowledged leaders in their fields and the topics are unique. Almost without exception, no other similar books exist on these topics.

Our goal is to publish books in important and rapidly changing areas of bioscience and environment for sophisticated researchers and clinicians. To achieve this goal, we have accelerated our publishing program to conform to the fast pace in which information grows in bioscience. Most of our books are published within 90 to 120 days of receipt of the manuscript. We would like to thank our readers for their continuing interest and welcome any comments or suggestions they may have for future books.

Shyamali Ghosh
Publications Director
R.G. Landes Company

CONTENTS

PREFACE

In industrialized countries, ischemic heart disease is by far the most common organ-specific cause of death. The thrombotic occlusion of a coronary artery which had previously been severely altered by atherosclerosis is the most frequent cause of acute myocardial infarction. Acute myocardial infarction still has a high mortality rate. Even if the patient survives the acute phase, the morbidity and long-term mortality are high. Myocardial infarction is the most frequent cause of heart failure which has a poor prognosis. Therefore, the immediate initiation of adequate diagnostic and therapeutic procedures is of vital consequence to the patient. Considerable progress has been made in therapeutic modalities to reperfuse ischemic myocardial tissue and to limit infarct size. However this is a double edged situation because the reliability of the diagnosis increases with the elapsed time from the onset of infarction, whereas in the interim the process of necrosis may progress. Consequently the induction of successful therapeutic measures depends to an increasing extent on early diagnostic results in a time frame of 4-6 hours after onset. To fulfill this demand, sensitive and reliable diagnostic tools are a prerequisite to optimize the efficacy of the therapeutic measures. However, the early sensitivities of the conventional laboratory markers for the diagnosis of myocardial damage (creatine kinase and lactate dehydrogenase isoenzymes) are too low to significantly contribute to the early diagnosis of infarction. During recent years a number of new markers with higher early sensitivities than aspartate aminotransferase, creatine kinase and lactate dehydrogenase activities have been proposed for the early diagnosis of myocardial infarction (for example, myoglobin, creatine kinase isoforms, creatine kinase MB mass concentration). At present there is enthusiasm that these markers will better meet the demands of clinicians. Another breakthrough in the diagnosis of myocardial damage was the introduction of sensitive and highly specific assays for measurement of cardiac troponin I and troponin T which will presumably become the criterion standard for diagnosis in patients with concomitant skeletal muscle damage. This book wants to satisfy the demand for a compilation of the current literature on new laboratory markers for myocardial injury and their application in clinical practice, and in this book, an attempt has been made to give a critical overview of current knowledge. The historical background of measurement of cardiac enzymes for diagnosis of myocardial damage is given in the introduction. The next chapter outlines the clinical significance of biochemical markers in the diagnosis of acute myocardial injury. Based on the limitations of the current standard markers creatine kinase and lactate dehydrogenase isoenzymes, the features of an ideal marker are worked out. The biochemical background and clinical results of new markers are given. The next chapter deals with the pathophysiological basis of myocardial protein release after myocardial infarction and the route of proteins from heart to serum. The diagnostic utility of biochemical markers in various clinical settings, such as acute or perioperative myocardial infarction, unstable angina or nonischemic myocardial damage, is discussed critically in the context of other routine clinical investigations. Finally, based on the literature results and own experience with new biochemical markers we offer guidelines. It is the hope of the authors that this stimulates the cost-effective use of myocardial markers in the routine laboratory in daily clinical practice.

CHAPTER 1

INTRODUCTION:
HISTORICAL BACKGROUND

The reports of Karmen et al[1] and of Ladue et al[2] in 1954 that serum aspartate aminotransferase (AST) activity was increased in patients with acute myocardial infarction (AMI) drew attention to enzymes as markers for myocardial damage and stimulated a vast increase in laboratory testing for AMI. In 1955, serum lactate dehydrogenase (LDH) activity was also found to be elevated after AMI.[3] The subsequent discovery that LDH activity in serum could be resolved into several fractions by electrophoresis improved the reliability of enzyme diagnosis of AMI considerably.[4] After AMI the fastest migrating fraction (LDH isoenzyme 1) was predominately found in serum, and LDH isoenzyme determination replaced AST for confirmation of myocardial injury because of greater heart-specificity.[5] In 1960 an increase in serum creatine kinase (CK) activity was first reported,[6] subsequently it was discovered that measurement of CK isoenzyme MB increases specificity and sensitivity for AMI.[7,8] Methods for the determination of CKMB isoenzyme became available for the routine hospital laboratory.[9,10] The more rapid appearance of CK in serum after AMI[7] and the high specificity for myocardial injury provided by determination of CKMB quickly established CKMB as the marker of choice for verifying suspected myocardial damage and measurement of CK and CKMB activity became the laboratory standard for excluding or confirming the diagnosis of AMI. However, it became soon clear that the electrocardiogram (ECG) could be normal despite biochemical evidence of myocardial injury and vice versa.[11] The World Health Organization (WHO) soon recognized the fundamental role of cardiac enzymes for the diagnosis of AMI and included the increase in cardiac enzymes as one criterion for the

diagnosis of AMI into its AMI criteria for the epidemiological studies on coronary artery disease by 1962.[12] Since then the increase
in cardiac enzymes remained one of three main criteria for diagnosis of definite AMI in all subsequent studies.[13] Accordingly, a
typical rising and falling pattern of CKMB alone in the proper
clinical setting is sufficient for AMI confirmation.[13] Although CK
and its isoenzyme MB have served for nearly three decades as criterion standard for the laboratory diagnosis of myocardial damage,
increases in CKMB are not as heart-specific as first believed, and
therefore, alternative, possibly more specific markers have been
investigated. Cardiac contractile and regulatory proteins gained
particular interest. Radioimmunoassays for measurement of cardiac
myosin light chain (MLC) were the first assays for cardiac contractile proteins to be reported in the literature.[14] Later on assays
for myosin heavy chains (MHC), tropomyosin, cardiac troponin I
(cTnI) and cardiac troponin T (cTnT) were developed.[15-18] Due to
complex and overlapping expression in human heart and skeletal
muscle cardiac MLC, MHC, and tropomyosin are not as heart-
specific as at first postulated, and, therefore, only the commercial-
ization of a cardiac-specific cTnT assay was a diagnostic breakthrough for the diagnosis of myocardial damage in routine clinical
practice. Recently, cardiac-specific cTnI assays have also bceome
commercially available. Therefore, it is necessary and the scope of
this book is to define the significance of these and other new biochemical markers for the diagnosis of myocardial damage in daily
clinical practice and to redefine the significance of the well-established commonly used markers CK and LDH isoenzymes.

REFERENCES

1. Karmen A, Wroblewski F, LaDue JS. Transaminase activity in human blood. J Clin Invest 1954; 34:126-33.
2. Ladue JS, Wroblewski F, Karmen A. Serum glutamic oxaloacetic
   transaminase activity in human acute myocardial infarction. Science 1954; 120:497-9.
3. Vessell ES, Bearn AG. Lactic dehydrogenase activity in blood. Proc
   Soc Exp Biol Med 1955; 90:210-3.
4. Vessel ES, Bearn AG. Localization of lactic acid dehydrogenase activity in serum fractions. Proc Soc Exp Biol Med 1957; 94:96-9.
5. Vasudevan G, Mercer DW, Varat MA. Lactic dehydrogenase isoenzyme determination in the diagnosis of acute myocardial infarction.
   Am J Cardiol 1978; 57:1055-7.

6. Dreyfus JC, Schapira G, Resnais J et al. La creatine-kinase serique dans le diagnostic de l'infarctus myocardique. Rev Fr Clin Biol 1960; 5:386-7.

7. Van der Veen KJ, Willebrands AF. Isoenzymes of creatine phosphokinase in tissue extracts and in normal and pathological sera. Clin Chim Acta 1966; 13:312-6.

8. Roberts R, Gowda KS, Ludbrook PA et al. Specificity of elevated serum MB creatine phosphokinase activity in the diagnosis of acute myocardial infarction. Am J Cardiol 1975; 36:433-7.

9. Roe CR, Limbird LE, Wagner GS et al. Combined isoenzyme analysis in the diagnosis of myocardial injury: application of electrophoretic methods for the detection and quantification of creatine kinase MB isoenzyme. J Lab Clin Med 1972; 80:577-90.

10. Neumeier D, Prellwitz W, Würzburg U et al. Determination of creatine kinase isoenzyme MB activity in serum using immunological inhibition of creatine kinase M subunit activity. Clin Chim Acta 1976; 73:445-51.

11. Pozen MD, D'Agostino RB, Selker HP et al. A predictive instrument to improve coronary care units admission practices in acute ischemic heart disease: a prospective multicenter clinical trial. New Engl J Med 1984; 310:1273-8.

12. Arterial Hypertension and ischemic heart disease. WHO Tech Rep Ser 1962; 231:18.

13. Tunstall-Pedoe H, Kuulasmaa K, Amouyel P et al. (WHO MONICA Project). Myocardial Infarction and coronary death in the World Health Organization MONICA Project—Registration procedures, event rates, and case fatality rates in 38 populations from 21 countries in 4 continents. Circulation 1994; 90:583-611.

14. Gere JB, Krauth GH, Trahern CA et al. A radioimmunoassay for the measurement of human cardiac myosin light chains. Am J Clin Pathol 1979; 71:309-18.

15. Leger JOC, Bouvagnet B, Pau B et al. Levels of ventricular myosin fragments in human sera after myocardial infarction, determined with monoclonal antibodies to myosin heavy chains. Eur J Clin Invest 1985; 15: 422-9.

16. Cummins P, McGurk B, Littler WA. Radioimmunoassay of human cardiac tropomyosin in acute myocardial infarction. Clin Science 1981; 60: 251-9.

17. Cummins B, Auckland ML, Cummins P. Cardiac-specific troponin I radioimmunoassay in the diagnosis of acute myocardial infarction. Am Heart J 1987; 113:1333-44.

18. Katus HA, Remppis A, Looser S et al. Enzyme linked immuno assay of cardiac troponin T for the detection of acute myocardial infarction in patients. J Mol Cell Cardiol 1989; 21:1349-53.

======= CHAPTER 2 =======

CLINICAL BACKGROUND:
THE CLINICAL SIGNIFICANCE OF BIOCHEMICAL MARKERS FOR DIAGNOSING ACUTE MYOCARDIAL DAMAGE

This chapter briefly summarizes the clinical background against which the hospital's laboratory has to deliver an efficient, cost-effective diagnostic service for the diagnosis of acute myocardial injury in cardiac diseases.

CORONARY ARTERY DISEASE

ACUTE MYOCARDIAL INFARCTION (AMI)

Pathogenesis

Myocardial ischemia as a consequence of coronary artery disease is the most frequent cause of acute myocardial damage. The pathogenesis of coronary artery disease has been extensively reviewed earlier (see refs. 1-4). Apart from reducing blood flow by reducing the patent cross section of a coronary artery, atheroma accretion also leads to an abnormal vasomotion of the atheromatous arterial wall which may react abnormally (increase in the severity of vasoconstriction) to neurogenic, paracrine or shear stresses. By plaque rupture and thrombosis a mild or moderate atheromatous lesion becomes a potential dangerous substrate for vessel obstruction. The clotting and thrombolytic processes are in a state of interaction and the final result depends on whether the thrombotic events are more active than thrombolysis. If partial occlusion results, it impairs blood flow and is manifested as unstable angina pectoris. Total obstruction leads to cessation of blood flow and, in most cases, acute myocardial infarction (AMI) occurs. Emboli from the local clot may also block distal coronary arteries. In approximately 50% of patients, the artery is obstructed abruptly. In the others, occlusion and dissolution occur, triggering a stuttering onset of complete occlusion, which is accompanied by antecedent warning signs, such as chest pain and T-wave changes in electrocardiography (ECG). Myocardial damage is a time-dependent process. Reimer and Jennings described the wave-front theory of AMI, in which subendocardial necrosis begins within 20 minutes and transmural infarction is complete within 4 hours.[5] This process can be modified, if the ischemic zone has a functioning collateral circulation, if conditioning had occurred, or if the artery opens and closes intermittently. This principal possibility to modify the process of myocardial necrosis development is the basis of all therapeutic interventions with the aim to reopen the infarct-related coronary artery and thereby minimizing irreversible myocardial damage and reducing early as well as long-term mortality and morbidity.[6] The process of AMI may be aborted if reperfusion is initiated within 30-40 minutes.

Diagnosis

Accurate early diagnosis of AMI is a prerequisite for proper triage and treatment, its clinical significance and modalities have been recently reviewed by Rozenman and Gotsman from a cardiologist's point of view.[7] Studies show that about 15% of all patients screened for new chest pain will develop AMI.[7] The most important diseases which have to be considered in the differential diagnosis of chest pain are listed in Table 2.1. Early diagnosis should be sensitive, so that all suitable patients can receive reperfusion therapy, and it must be specific as well, so that patients without AMI are not exposed to unnecessary risks of reperfusion therapy. Triage in the emergency department should accurately predict, whether the patient must be admitted to the coronary care unit, should have a monitored bed, can be admitted to a general medical ward, or may be discharged with additional investigations as an outpatient.

The diagnosis of a large AMI in a previously symptomless patient with typical risk factors (a history of a prior AMI or sys-

Table 2.1. Differential diagnoses for chest pain

1. Cardiovascular diseases
   - Coronary artery disease (myocardial infarction, angina pectoris)
   - Pericarditis
   - Aortic aneurysm / dissection
   - Congestive heart failure
   - Aortic stenosis
   - Hypertrophic obstructive cardiomyopathy
   - Mitral valve prolapse
   - Mediastinitis
   - Heart contusion
   - Postmyocardial infarction (Dressler's) syndrome

2. Pulmonary diseases
   - Pneumonia
   - Pulmonary embolism
   - Pneumothorax
   - Pleurisy
   - Pulmonary hypertension

3. Gastrointestinal diseases
   - Peptic ulcer disease
   - Acute cholecystitis
   - Pancreatitis
   - Gastroesophageal reflux / esophagitis
   - Esophageal spasm

4. Neurologic diseases
   - Dermatomal sensory abnormalities
   - Herpes zoster dermatitis

5. Muskuloskeletal Diseases
   - Rib fractures / chest contusion
   - Costochondral and chondrosternal disorders
   - Intercostal muscle cramping
   - Shoulder / clavicular bursitis and tendinitis
   - Cervical arthritis
   - Cervical disk rupture

6. Anxiety states

7. Cocaine abuse induced chest pain

temic atherosclerosis, family history of premature coronary artery disease, smoking addiction, dyslipidemia, adipositas, hypertension, diabetes, or age over 70 years) seldom presents a significant problem to the clinician. The diagnosis of an AMI is generally based upon the presence of at least two out of three classic findings: i.e., clinical history of ischemic chest discomfort of more than

20 minutes duration (does not respond to nitroglycerin), the evolution of typical, unequivocal electrocardiographic changes (definite abnormal Q waves or equivalents) in at least 2 leads of the 12-lead standard ECG, and the rise and fall of serum enzymes indicative of myocardial muscle fiber injury.[6-9]

History and symptoms

Typical clinical symptoms include prolonged pressing, squeezing and burning chest pain, which is usually retrosternal, but may radiate or can occur in the lower jaw, back, arms, shoulders, wrist or epigastrium with or without symptoms of excessive autonomic nervous system activity (e.g., nausea, vomiting, cold perspiration). AMI patients are usually anxious and distressed. The physical signs vary depending on the size of infarction and its hemodynamic consequences and range from minimal hemodynamic disturbance to pulmonary edema and cardiogenic shock. A patient with chest pain that can be elicited by chest-wall palpation is less likely to have an AMI, but this finding is for several reasons not wholly reliable. Although most patients present with typical symptoms, myocardial ischemia, even when prolonged, is not always accompanied by chest pain. As many as one in three AMIs is not clinically recognized by either patient or physician because the chest pain is atypical or absent,[10,11] and physicians send home from emergency departments one of every 20 patients with AMI. Common reasons for missing the diagnosis AMI are listed in Table 2.2. The incidence of silent myocardial infarction is higher in diabetic patients[12] and appears to be more common in women than men.[10] It is noteworthy that particularly in the elderly AMI frequently present atypically. On the other hand, many patients who present with typical symptoms have unstable angina.

Electrocardiography (ECG)

The medical history is a valuable source for diagnosing AMI, but the diagnosis should be confirmed by ECG. The ECG is a simple, convenient, reliable and reproducible method for early diagnosis. Diagnostic early changes include regional ST-segment elevation which is often preceded by changes in the T wave (peaked T wave) and a widened QRS complex. Occasionally only ST-segment depression or T wave inversion appears. ST-T segment depression is very nonspecific and also frequently occurs with tran-

Table 2.2. Common reasons for missing the diagnosis of acute myocardial infarction

1. Obtaining an "atypical" history

2. Assuming that a patient is too young for suffering an acute myocardial infarction

3. Semantic misunderstandings between physician and patient

4. Undue reliance on the absence of cardiac risk factors

5. Ascribing all chest wall pain as being musculoskeletal in origin or erroneously interpreting chest pain produced by palpation as the same as patient's original complaint

6. Misinterpreting or relying on normal electrocardiograms

7. Inappropriate use and interpretation of serum cardiac marker results (relying on negative test results at times too early after the onset of chest pain to rule out myocardial infarction, choosing markers incorrectly)

8. Using too narrow criteria for admitting and monitoring patients (using drugs, such as nitroglycerin and antacids, to rule myocardial infarction in or out, missing a second chance to make the diagnosis during follow-up care)

sient reversible ischemia. In rare cases no changes are found.[13] Unfortunately, unequivocal clinical symptoms and ECG findings are not present or easily discerned in every AMI patient. ECG findings in patients with presumed AMI are often unresolved. Early ECG findings in the setting of evolving AMI are frequently nondiagnostic. Some changes are subtle and even experienced electrocardiographers have difficulty deciding whether they result from cardiac ischemia. This is true in particular for non-Q wave AMI (see below). When only the admission ECG is considered in patients with prolonged chest pain and no prior infarction, the overall diagnostic efficiency is 75%.[14] Retrospective assessment of serial ECGs—by which time it may be too late for therapeutic interventions—increases the efficiency to 94%.[15] Nonetheless, the ECG is misleading in at least 8% of all AMIs and is indeterminate in an additional 12% of patients, primarily because of the presence of an abnormal baseline ECG (e.g., left bundle branch block, other conduction disturbances, ventricular pacemaker, previous infarction with persistent ST-segment elevation) or nonspecific ST-T wave abnormalities.[15] Many other problems, such as infection, inflammation, aneurysms, early repolarization and hyperkalemia may mimic ECG patterns otherwise indicative of AMI. Nearly 50% of patients with AMI will initially have nondiagnostic ECGs on emergency department presentation.[16] When ST-segment elevation was the diagnostic criterion, the sensitivity for AMI was 50-60% and the specificity 90-95%, respectively.[17-19] When any other acute ischemic changes are included in the criteria, the sensitivity increases to about 70%, but the specificity drops to approximately 50%. Diagnostic accuracy increases if the ECG is examined in conjunction with the patient's detailed medical history and a physical examination.[17] Only a small percentage of patients with normal ECG and only a vague clinical suspicion of AMI suffered infarction. On the other hand, patients with typical risk factors, a typical clinical presentation and ECG changes do not present a diagnostic dilemma. However, in the high-suspicion group only about one third actually develop AMI, and clearly additional tests must be performed on this patient group to increase diagnostic specificity. Thus, clinical history and ECG changes fail to diagnose AMI accurately in an important minority of AMI patients.

Myocardial infarctions are subdivided into two groups (Q wave and non-Q wave AMI), based on whether or not new definitive abnormal Q waves develop in the patient's ECG.[20] The ECG observations should be reported as such and the formerly used terms transmural and subendocardial AMI should not be used any longer, because it has become apparent that there is only a poor correlation between the ECG findings and the actual tissue pathology. The presence or absence of Q waves on the surface ECG does not necessarily identify anatomically transmural or nontransmural AMI, because transmural infarctions may have no Q waves and vice versa. There are important differences between uncomplicated Q wave and non-Q wave AMIs; they differ physiologically and clinically.[20] About 40% of AMIs occurring are non-Q wave. The in-hospital mortality is higher for Q wave AMIs, but the longer term mortalities of both are identical. Non-Q wave AMIs more frequently develop postinfarct unstable angina or reinfarction than Q wave AMIs, because of a larger residual mass of viable but jeopardized myocardium within the perfusion zone of the infarct-related vessel. Therefore coronary angioplasty or bypass graft surgery are frequently needed in these patients. An occluded infarct-related coronary artery is found in up to 90% of Q wave AMIs,[21] but in only up to 20% of non-Q wave AMIs.[20,22] Non-Q wave AMIs usually undergo early spontaneous reperfusion. Therefore, in contrast to Q wave AMIs the benefits of reperfusion therapy are not clearly established in non-Q wave AMIs. In the latter, pharmacologically induced thrombolysis after 2-3 hours may be redundant, since reperfusion has already occurred. Non-Q wave AMIs are characterized by smaller infarct size presumably due to early reperfusion as a result of spontaneous thrombolysis, a relief of vasospasm, or both, and a better left ventricular function, unless impaired by previous AMI.

The diagnosis of non-Q wave AMI may be suspected from ECG findings but must be confirmed by enzyme determinations or other clinical investigations. In non-Q wave AMI, the ECG abnormalities are nonspecific (70-80% present with ST segment depression) and have to be taken into account with the clinical picture as infarction cannot be established with certainty in the absence of alterations of the QRS complex.

Other noninvasive diagnostic techniques for early myocardial infarction diagnosis

Noninvasive diagnostic imaging techniques, such as myocardial scintigraphy or echocardiography, are important tools for assessment and management of AMI. However, they are unlikely to help in the early diagnosis of AMI in the immediate future because of either expense, practical feasibility, or difficulty of interpretation.[7,23]

Nuclear studies: Technetium-99m pyrophosphate scintigraphy is too insensitive for early AMI diagnosis. Antimyosin antibody imaging remains investigational at present and is not more sensitive either. Thallium-201 and technetium setamibi myocardial scintigraphy certainly provide valuable information for the management of chest pain patients, but both detect ischemia and cannot distinguish it from necrosis. Perfusion defects do not distinguish between acute ischemia, AMI, or previous infarction. These diagnostic techniques are mostly not available on a 24 hour a day basis and are not clinically applicable for widespread screening, they are expensive and do not discriminate between old and new injury. Radionuclide ventriculography for detection of regional wall motion abnormalities offers some potential. It has the limitations of myocardial scintigraphy, but is less sensitive and specific. Echocardiography is more suitable for the evaluation of the emergency room patient with chest pain to assess wall motion.

Fast cine computerized tomography, magnetic resonance imaging, and positron emission tomography are all too cumbersome for early diagnosis and it is unlikely that they will be applied in the near future, because they are either too insensitive to detect early changes, too expensive, or time consuming.

Echocardiography: A significant advantage of this technique is that it can be performed at the bedside or in the emergency room and results are immediately available and relatively easy to interpret.[24,25] Faced with an atypical clinical chart, emergency cardiac echocardiography is important for ruling out pericarditis or aortic dissection. However, good equipment and experience in the interpretation of echocardiographic results are mandatory for reliable AMI diagnosis. Immediately after coronary occlusion, the myocardium ceases to function in the area of the infarct-related vessel. On echocardiography regional wall motion abnormalities can be detected (e.g., hypokinesia, akinesia, dyskinesia, systolic wall thickening disappears, the wall may even thin during systole). This is a sensitive index because the lack of function occurs rapidly after myocardial ischemia. However, large studies to evaluate the diagnostic accuracy of echocardiography for early AMI detection are still missing and warranted.[23] Echocardiography cannot distinguish between old and new injury (preexisting and new wall motion abnormalities) and regional wall-motion abnormalities are less common in patients with non-Q wave AMI. A segmentic kinetics disorder, suggesting AMI, can also be the result of severe myocardial ischemia, repeated or prolonged, but without myocardial necrosis (stunned or hibernating myocardium). Another limitation is inadequate images that occur in 5-10% of patients.[23]

Significance of biochemical markers

From all the limitations of the different diagnostic procedures outlined above it is clear that undoubtedly there is a role of biochemical markers for diagnosis of AMI. Serum levels of intramyocardial proteins are easier to interpret than ECG, echocardiography and all the other imaging techniques. Biochemical markers are the most accurate means of diagnosing AMI. Modern medical practice requires rapid decisions in AMI patients. Clinicians demand rapid assays that are simple to perform and markers should accurately accomplish several goals: (1) differentiate patients with and without AMI early after the onset of symptoms for a more effective triaging in the emergency room and possibly a more cost effective use of intensive care beds; (2) distinguish patients who have coronary recanalization after treatment with thrombolytic agents from those who do not, so that those in need of additional treatment can be identified and unnecessary cardiac catheterization may be prevented and (3) permit estimation of infarct size, a reliable predictor of survival after AMI.[26]

However, as will be discussed in detail in the next chapter, in patients with concomitant skeletal muscle damage (e.g., postoperative or traumatized patients, or after cardiopulmonary resuscitation) the diagnostic efficiency of creatine kinase (CK) MB and lactate dehydrogenase (LDH) isoenzyme-1 is limited. Increases in CKMB occur too late for optimal early AMI diagnosis or prompt detection of coronary recanalization. The sensitivity of a combination of CK, LDH and aspartate aminotransferase (AST) for patients in the early stages of an AMI is only 20-30%. In addition, the complex kinetics of CKMB release after reperfusion hampers analysis of infarct size. At present there is enthusiasm that new biochemical markers will better meet the demands of the cardiologist.

PERIOPERATIVE MYOCARDIAL INFARCTION

Noncardiac surgery

The incidence of perioperative myocardial infarction (PMI) with noncardiac surgery varies by the type of procedure and the prevalence of coronary atherosclerosis in the study population. Incidence is ≤1% with minor procedures and may exceed 10% with vascular operations. As surgical techniques have become increasingly sophisticated, the percentage of perioperative morbidity and mortality attributable to other complications rather than direct surgical problems has grown. Myocardial infarction is a common cause of morbidity and mortality in patients who had noncardiac surgery.[27] The mortality among patients with PMI is high ranging from 30-50%.[28,29] In particular, patients requiring vascular surgery are at risk to develop PMI because this group has a high incidence of coronary artery disease, which increases the risk of PMI.

To minimize cardiac risk in noncardiac surgery, the clinician must estimate preoperatively the individual risk for PMI development and must be able to detect PMI and treat its complications. The modalities of diagnosis are the same as for AMI, however it is more difficult to diagnose PMI for the following reasons: symptoms of ischemia or infarction are uncommon perioperatively.[27] Because of the effects of medications (anesthesia, analgesics), most PMI patients do not note chest pain[30] or pain may be difficult to be attributed to the heart. In addition, a high frequency of notable but apparently innocent postoperative ECG changes limits the diagnostic use of ECG. Metabolic abnormalities can mask ECG findings. Approximately 20% of preoperative ECGs and an additional 25% of postoperative ECGs are uninterpretable.[27] Many episodes of perioperative ischemia which is assumed to be often a precursor of PMI occur without changes in heart rate or blood pressure.[31] Most of the above mentioned imaging techniques for detection of AMI are too cumbersome or can be hardly performed in the early postoperative period when intensive care monitoring is necessary, and only transthoracic and particularly transoesophageal two-dimensional echocardiography is important means of diagnosing PMI. However, as mentioned above, small myocardial infarctions need not necessarily lead to segmental-wall motion abnormalities and may be missed. Therefore, biochemical markers could play a major role in PMI diagnosis. Their use should be simpler and more cost effective than the routine use of echocardiography. To diagnose PMI in noncardiac surgery patients, diagnostic strategies should be similar to those used with patients not having surgery, with special emphasis on serial sampling and using the CKMB/CK ratio to distinguish noncardiac from cardiac sources of increased CKMB to reduce false positive results.[30] In practice the CKMB/CK ratio has low sensitivity and variable specificity for cardiac injury in surgical patients, and sometimes a PMI cannot be diagnosed with certainty or excluded based on CKMB measurements. Assays for LDH isoenzymes are less useful because LDH-1 is not heart-specific and, for example, hemolysis associated with surgical trauma can cause an isoenzyme profile similar to that of myocardial infarction. Consequently a serum marker with a higher specificity than CKMB and as high a sensitivity is highly desirable and would facilitate the detection and treatment of PMI, which would help to define the significance of PMI for prognosis.

Cardiac surgery

Regarding the development of PMI, coronary artery bypass grafting (CABG) is the most relevant surgical procedure. CABG is a procedure that bypasses several stenoses of coronary arteries with a grafted segment of the patient's own saphenous vein or internal mammary artery. Cardiopulmonary bypass (extracorporal circulation) with cardioplegia and aortic crossclamping and systemic and topical cardiac hypothermia are frequently used to maintain the circulation while rendering the heart bloodless and immobile for CABG surgery. CABG carries a risk of PMI. PMI remains a major and frequent complication following CABG and adversely affects prognosis.[32,33] Reports of its incidence vary from 5% to 35% (on average 5-10%). Although CABG patients can expect a subsequent reduction in risk of developing postoperative ischemia, they are at the same time at an increased risk of developing perioperative ischemia compared to noncardiac surgical patients. Extensive Q wave PMI are reliably detected by ECG and CKMB measurements. Apart from large myocardial infarction, the diagnosis of PMI is difficult because there is no classic presentation. The diagnostic modalities and their limitations are the same as in PMI after noncardiac surgery with special emphasis on the important roles of ECG and echocardiography. Many perturbations of various potential diagnostic criteria are related not only to myocardial infarction but also to the surgical procedure, cardioplegia, hypothermia, hemolysis and other factors. Consequently, the reliability of every criterion used for the diagnosis of small PMI—ECG, myocardial scintigraphy, echocardiography, and enzyme changes— has limitations. Several authors[30,32] recommend the confirmation of at least two positive criteria (ECG, myocardial scintigraphy, development of new regional wall motion abnormalities, or enzyme results) as evidence of PMI.

Both clinical symptoms and ECG changes have inherent limitations. Therefore, biochemical markers for myocardial injury are critical diagnostic tools. However, after CABG the significance of the usual reference limits of enzyme concentration in serum are invalid as a consequence of inevitable cardiac (e.g., cardioplegia, cannulation with right atriotomy) and extracardiac tissue damage occurring during the surgical procedure. The interpretation of CKMB elevation is made considerably more complex. Only increases in CKMB of more than 12-18 hours duration correlate well with other evidence for myocardial infarction.[30] Assays for LDH isoenzymes are less useful because hemolysis associated with surgical trauma and extracorporal circulation can cause an isoenzyme profile similar to that of myocardial infarction. Nonetheless, carefully analyzed serial serum marker data can yield diagnostically useful information, but sensitive and more cardiac-specific markers are needed.

UNSTABLE ANGINA PECTORIS

Unstable angina is common and often quite serious and causes significant disability and death in industrialized countries.[34,35] The overall 1 year mortality (approximately 10%) is about one-third that of AMI patients, but there is a high-risk subgroup. Patients with unstable angina represent a heterogeneous group. Unstable angina pectoris is a transitory clinical syndrome intermediate between chronic, stable (exertional) angina which is usually predictable by the patient and AMI. The natural history is typically characterized by either progression to nonfatal AMI or death or by resumption to chronic stable angina. Patients without unstable angina during at least 1 week before AMI are rare. Unstable angina pectoris comprises patients with accelerated angina (preexisting stable angina with progressive and prolonged angina), new onset angina, or patients with acute or subacute chest pain at rest or provoked by minimal exertion.[34,35] Class I of the Braunwald classifications (accelerated angina) comprises patients with new onset of severe or accelerated angina without pain at rest, class II (subacute angina at rest) angina at rest within past month but not within the preceding 48 hours, and class III (acute angina at rest) angina at rest within 48 hours, respectively. According to clinical circumstances unstable angina is subdivided into secondary unstable angina (class A, angina developed due to extracardiac conditions), primary unstable angina (class B), and postinfarction unstable angina (class C) shortly after myocardial infarction (within 2 weeks). Asymptomatic patients or patients with stable angina for more than 2 month are not considered as suffering unstable angina. Both increased myocardial oxygen demand in presence of severely restricted coronary reserve and dynamic stenosis caused by coronary vasoconstriction may be responsible for unstable angina. Rapid progression of coronary stenosis often precedes the development of unstable angina. The stenosis is frequently eccentric and often associated with coronary thrombi. Variant (Prinzmetal's) angina is a subtype of unstable angina at rest with ECG changes (ST-segment elevation). It is not precipitated by exertion or stress, it is due to focal coronary artery spasm. In most but not all patients with unstable angina symptoms are caused by coronary artery disease. Typically the coronary artery that has ruptured at one side shows atherosclerotic plaques and a fresh thrombus that does not necessarily occlude the vessel. Secondary unstable angina may be caused by diseases that reduce the myocardial oxygen supply (e.g., anemia) or increase the myocardial oxygen demand (e.g., thyrotoxicosis). The clinical symptoms may be accompanied by ST segment or T wave alterations in the ECG. In the latter subgroup of patients a release of myocardial fiber constituents can be expected due to ischemic cell damage. Histologic findings (cell swelling, small areas of necrosis) indicate minor myocardial necrosis in high-risk patients with unstable angina. These patients do not meet the standard enzymatic and ECG criteria for myocardial infarction. Only if the area of myocardial necrosis is large enough to be detected by ECG changes or by the use of conventional cardiac enzyme criteria, then myocardial infarction is diagnosed. Therefore, the distinction between small non-Q wave infarction and unstable angina pectoris is only a shade of gray. For appropriate therapy and preventive measures the challenge is not always simply to rule in or rule out myocardial infarction, but rather to distinguish patients with acutely unstable coronary lesions from those with either stable coronary disease or none. The lack of sensitivity of CK and CKMB activity and LDH isoenzyme assays makes it very difficult to determine whether or not small amounts of myocardial necrosis are present in patients with chest pain. A small rise in serum CK activity occurs in some patients. However, CKMB activities stay within the reference interval in most patients. Diagnostic markers of high sensitivity and specificity must be employed for the detection of this limited myocardial injury. Recently, a much higher percentage of patients with unstable angina and increased CKMB in blood was described by measuring CKMB as mass concentration using immunometric CKMB assays.[36,37] Compared to patients with stable angina, those with unstable angina have an increased risk of AMI and death.[38] Many patients with unstable angina do not develop serious complications, but among these patients a high-risk subgroup may be identified. Several parameters, such as persisting or recurring chest pain, rapid development of symptoms, ST-segment and T wave changes on the ECG, perfusion abnormalities in myocardial scintigraphy, reduced left ventricular function or extensive coronary artery disease, have been used for identification of this high-risk subgroup,[38-42] but more reliable noninvasive methods are needed to select patients for urgent cardiac catheterization.[43] To prevent the eventual development of AMI in patients with unstable angina, it is, therefore, also desirable to find a laboratory parameter with higher sensitivity and specificity than CKMB which efficiently identifies patients at risk to develop myocardial infarction.[43] This marker should not be detectable in patients without myocardial damage.

NONISCHEMIC MYOCARDIAL DAMAGE

MYOCARDITIS

Acute myocarditis has a highly variable presentation and clinical course, which presents the clinician with a difficult diagnostic and prognostic challenge. The natural history of myocarditis is highly variable. Mostly the disease is self-limited without causing further sequelea. However, antiarrhythmic therapy or pacemaker implantation may be necessary. In patients who develop acute dilated cardiomyopathy, the disease may proceed to chronic dilated cardiomyopathy and progressive heart failure. Although the clinical manifestations of myocarditis may alert the physician to the illness, endomyocardial biopsy is necessary to confirm the diagnosis.[44-46] But this technique has limitations related to sampling errors, and a negative result does not necessarily exclude myocarditis. In general, histology has been of limited value to predict clinical outcome. The therapeutic approach to patients with confirmed myocarditis remains controversial, especially with respect to the use of immunosuppressive agents. Noninvasive markers for identifying, at the time of presentation, high-risk patients who may benefit from aggressive therapy are of great interest.

Myocarditis can be caused by a number of infectious (viruses, bacteria, spirochetes, fungal, rickettsia, parasites) and noninfectious agents (e.g., toxic, radiation, chemical and drug effects, hypersensitivity, rejection of the transplanted heart). Myocarditis may also be a manifestation of a systemic illness, such as vasculitis or sarcoidosis. In North America and Europe viruses are the most common agents producing myocarditis.[45,46] The most common causes are enteroviruses, especially Coxackie B. The mechanism by which viral infection results in myocardial necrosis and inflammation is not entirely known. The initial myocardial injury is caused by the virus itself, but the ongoing myocardial inflammation is probably secondary to an immunoresponse against myocardial surface antigens altered by the viral infection.[45]

Since detection of virus-neutralizing antibodies in serum is only useful for retrospective diagnosis, the diagnosis of myocarditis is based mainly on clinical signs and symptoms. A high index of suspicion is often necessary. The clinical presentation shows wide variations, ranging from a total absence of clinical manifestations to chest pain, symptoms and signs of heart failure, arrhythmias and conduction abnormalities, or sudden unexpected death.[44-46] It is likely that many patients with the condition are asymptomatic and never seek medical attention. The presence of myocarditis is often inferred from unspecific ECG abnormalities, particularly arrhythmias, disturbances of the conducting system, ST segment elevation, flattening or inversion of T waves. Although there are many noninvasive techniques that can provide evidence to support a diagnosis of myocarditis, right ventricular multiple endomyocardial biopsy is the criterion standard for confirmation of myocarditis against which all other tests are compared. Clinical characteristics in patients with suspected myocarditis have correlated poorly with histologic findings on biopsy.[47] Clinical characteristics, baseline hemodynamics and left ventricular ejection fraction are poor predictors of outcome. Gallium-67 nuclear imaging may be suitable for diagnosing and monitoring myocardial inflammation and antimyosin imaging may be a useful screening tool for the detection of myocardial necrosis in patients with suspected myocarditis, but these techniques need further evaluation.[46] Due to lack of sensitivity and specificity (as discussed earlier), measurements of CKMB and LDH-1 are often inconclusive as well. CK activities do not predict which patients will have evidence of myocardial inflammation and necrosis on biopsy.[47]

Despite various efforts to obtain diagnostic criteria and techniques, the diagnosis of "myocarditis" remains a diagnostic and prognostic dilemma in many cases.[48,49] The introduction of a sensitive and cardiac-specific marker of myocardial injury could bring a breakthrough in patients with myocarditis or cardiomyopathies.

BLUNT CARDIAC TRAUMA

Cardiac injury occurs commonly after blunt trauma with chest contusion, sudden deceleration/acceleration, or rapid increases in the intrathoracic pressure.[50] The true incidence is unknown. In patients with a history of blunt chest trauma, it varies from 5-75%, depending on the thoroughness of the diagnostic evaluation.[50] Nonpenetrating injuries of the heart (myocardial contusion) result from the effects of external physical forces and are frequently overlooked. They can be classified as being predominantly functional or anatomic in their manifestations with disruption of myocardial cells (cell necrosis and fragmentation), but there is a tremendous overlap. The consequences of nonpenetrating injury to the myocardium vary in intensity from mild contusion with subtle, subclinical wall motion or conduction abnormalities, which are frequently detectable only after intense investigations, to significant depression in ventricular function or pump failure, lethal arrhythmias or cardiac rupture which produces immediate death from pericardial tamponade or exsanguination.[50,51] Because of its location immediately posterior to the sternum, the right ventricle (small muscle mass) is the most frequently injured chamber.[50] Clinical manifestations also vary proportionately and a high index of suspicion is often necessary for their recognition in all but the most obvious cases. There are few reliable signs and symptoms that are specific for cardiac contusion. The clinical diagnosis of a heart contusion is generally based on a CKMB/CK activity index of more than 5% facultative together with ECG alterations (arrhythmias, conduction disturbances, ST-T segment alterations) or a positive result in two-dimensional echocardiography.[52] However, there are no well-defined and uniformly accepted criteria. A number of diagnostic techniques have additionally been tested in the diagnosis of heart contusion but there are no generally agreed upon criteria for the diagnosis of myocardial contusion in living humans. The reliability of all criteria used (e.g., ECG, technetium-labeled pyrophosphate scanning, thallium single-photon emission computed tomography [SPECT] scintigraphy, antimyosin scintigraphy, radionuclide angiography, echocardiography) is the subject of much discussion in the literature.[50,53,54] In particular, the value of CKMB measurements as a screening test for heart contusion in trauma victims has been questioned by recently published studies.[55,56] Even serial CKMB measurement lacks sensitivity as well as specificity. At present no single test or combination of tests has proven consistently reliable in detecting cardiac injury and clinical outcome thereby influencing significantly the management of asymptomatic patients suspected as having cardiac contusion.[50] Myocardial contusion may be only be diagnosed with certainty at autopsy or during thoracotomy. The prognosis of patients with myocardial contusion is difficult to discern. In general it appears to be excellent without long-term sequelae,[50] although sometimes in individual patients the development of septal defects or ventricular aneurysms and pseudoaneurysms may require surgical intervention. The introduction of a sensitive and cardiac-specific marker of myocardial injury with higher sensitivity and specificity than CKMB could certainly bring a breakthrough in the diagnosis of heart contusion and could help to better define the clinical significance of this disease and its prognostic implications in patients who do not immediately die from its complications (cardiac rupture).

REFERENCES

1. Fuster V, Badimon L, Badimon JJ et al. The pathogenesis of coronary artery disease and acute coronary syndromes. New Engl J Med 1991; 326:242-50.
2. Ross R. The pathogenesis of atherosclerosis-an update. New Engl J Med 1986; 314:488-500.
3. Davies MJ, Thomas AC. Plaque fissure-the cause of acute myocardial infarction, sudden ischemic death, and crescendo angina. Br Heart J 1985; 53:363-73.
4. Falk E. Coronary thrombosis: pathogenesis and clinical manifestations. Am J Cardiol 1991; 68:28B-35B.
5. Reimer KA, Jennings RB. The "wavefront phenomenon" of myocardial ischemic cell death. II. Transmural progression of necrosis within the frame work of ischemic bed size (myocardium at risk) and collateral flow. Lab Invest 1979; 40:633-44.
6. AHA Medical/Scientific Statement (special report): ACC/AHA Guidelines for the early management of patients with acute myocardial infarction. Circulation 1990; 82:664-707.
7. Rozenman Y, Gotsman MS. The earliest diagnosis of acute myocardial infarction. Annu Rev Med 1994; 45:31-44.
8. Tunstall-Pedoe H, Kuulasmaa K, Amouyel P et al. (WHO MONICA Project). Myocardial Infarction and coronary death in the World Health Organization MONICA Project—Registration procedures, event rates, and case fatality rates in 38 populations from 21 countries in 4 continents. Circulation 1994; 90:583-611.

9. Gillum RF, Fortmann SP, Prineas RJ et al. International diagnostic criteria for acute myocardial infarction and acute stroke. Am Heart J 1984; 108:150-8.

10. Kannel WB. Prevalence and clinical aspects of unrecognized myocardial infarction and sudden unexpected death. Circulation 1987; 75 (suppl II): II-4-5.

11. Grimm RH, Tillingshast S, Daniels K et al. Unrecognized myocardial infarction: experience in the multiple risk factor intervention trial (MRFIT). Circulation 1987; 75 (suppl II):II-6-8.

12. Gregoratos G. Management of uncomplicated acute myocardial infarction. In: Parmely WW and Chatterjee K, eds. Cardiology. Philadelphia, JB Lippincott Co, 1990, Vol. 2:10-7 - 10.

13. Timmis A. Early diagnosis of myocardial infarction: electrocardiography is still the best. Br Med J 1990; 301:941-2.

14. Rude RE, Poole WK, Muller JE et al. Electrocardiographic and clinical criteria for recognition of acute myocardial infarction based on analysis of 3697 patients. Am J Cardiol 1983; 52:936-42.

15. Turi ZG, Rutherford JD, Roberts R et al. Electrocardiographic, enzymatic and scintigraphic criteria of acute myocardial infarction as determined from study of 726 patients (a MILIS study). Am J Cardiol 1985; 55:1463-8.

16. Gibler WB, Lewis LM, Erb RE et al. Early detection of acute myocardial infarction in patients presenting with chest pain and nondiagnostic ECGs: serial CKMB sampling in the emergency department. Ann Emerg Med 1990; 19:1359-66.

17. Karlson BW, Herlitz J, Wiklund O et al. Early prediction of acute myocardial infarction from clinical history, examination, and electrocardiogram in the emergency room. Am J Cardiol 1991; 68:171-5.

18. Weaver WD, Eisenberg MS, Martin JS et al. Myocardial infarction triage and intervention project-phase I: patient characteristics and feasibility of prehospital initiation of thrombolytic therapy. J Am Coll Cardiol 1990; 15:925-31.

19. Kudenchuk PJ, Ho MT, Weaver WD et al. Accuracy of computer interpreted electrocardiography in selecting patients for thrombolytic therapy. J Am Coll Cardiol 1991; 17:1486-91.

20. Gibson RS. Non-Q-wave myocardial infarction: pathophysiology, prognosis, and therapeutic strategy. Annu Rev Med 1989; 40:395-410.

21. DeWood MA, Spores J, Notske R et al. Prevalence of total coronary occlusion during the early hours of transmural myocardial infarction. New Engl J Med 1980; 303:897-902.

22. Bren GB, Wasserman AG, Ross AM et al. TIMI Investigators. Coronary perfusion status in Q- and non-Q-wave infarction patients presenting with ST elevation (abstract). Circulation 1987; 76 (suppl IV): IV-123.

23. Roberts R, Kleiman NS. Earlier diagnosis and treatment of acute myocardial infarction necessitates the need for a "new diagnostic mind-set". Circulation 1994; 89:872-81.

24. Quinones MA, Roberts R. Role of two-dimensional echocardiography in acute myocardial infarction. Echocardiography 1985; 2:213-6.

25. Saiba P, Afrookteh A, Touchstone DA et al. Value of regional wall motion abnormality in emergency room diagnosis of acute myocardial infarction: a prospective study using two-dimensional echocardiography. Circulation 1991; 84(suppl I):I-85-I-92.

26. Geltman EM, Ehsani AA, Campbell MK et al. The influence of location and extent of myocardial infarction on long-term ventricular dysrhythmia and mortality. Circulation 1979; 60:805-14.

27. Mangano DT. Perioperative cardiac morbidity. Anesthesiology 1990; 72:153-84.

28. Roberts SL, Tinker JH. Cardiovascular disease, risk, and outcome in anesthesia. Philadelphia: JB Lippincott, 1988:33-49.

29. London MJ, Mangano DT. Assessment of perioperative risk. In: Stoelting RK, ed. Advances in anesthesia. Vol. 5, Chicago: Year Book Medical, 1988:53-87.

30. Lee TH, Goldman L. Serum enzyme assays in the diagnosis of acute myocardial infarction-recommendations based on a quantitative analysis. Ann Intern Med 1985; 105:221-33.

31. Mangano DT, Browner WS, Hollenberg M et al. Association of perioperative myocardial ischemia with cardiac morbidity and mortality in men undergoing noncardiac surgery. New Engl J Med 1990; 323:1781-8.

32. Force TH, Hibbert P, Weeks G et al. Perioperative myocardial infarction after coronary artery bypass surgery. Clinical significance and approach to risk stratification. Circulation 1990; 82, 903-12.

33. Jain U. Myocardial infarction during coronary artery bypass surgery (Review). J Cardiothorac Vasc Anesth 1992; 6:612-23.

34. Braunwald E. Unstable angina a classification. Circulation 1989; 80:410-4.

35. Braunwald E, Jones RH, Mark DB et al. Diagnosing and Managing unstable angina. Circulation 1994; 90:613-22.

36. Gerhardt W, Katus H, Ravkilde J et al. S-troponin T in suspected ischemic myocardial injury compared with mass and catalytic concentrations of S-creatine kinase isoenzyme MB. Clin Chem 1991; 37:1405-11.

37. Botker HE, Ravkilde J, Sogaard P et al. Gradation of unstable angina on the basis of a sensitive method for creatine kinase MB isoenzyme determination in serum. Br Heart J 1991; 65:72-6.

38. Gazes PC, Mobley EM, Faris HM et al. Preinfarction angina: a prospective study: ten years follow up. Prognostic significance of electrocardiographic changes. Circulation 1973; 48:331-7.

39. Freeman MR, Williams AE, Chisholm RJ et al. Role of resting thallium 201 perfusion in predicting coronary anatomy, left ventricular wall motion, and hospital outcome in unstable angina pectoris. Am Heart J 1989; 117:306-14.

40. Nordlander R, Nyquist O. Patients treated in a coronary care unit without acute myocardial infarction. Identification of high risk subgroup for subsequent myocardial infarction and/or cardiovascular death. Br Heart J 1979; 41:647-53.

41. Scarlovsky S, Rechavia E, Strasberg B et al. Unstable angina: ST segment depression with positive versus negative T wave deflections—clinical course, ECG evolution, and angiographic correlation. Am Heart J 1988; 116:933-41.

42. Betriu A, Heras M, Cohen M, Fuster V. Unstable angina: outcome according to clinical presentation. J Am Coll Cardiol 1992; 19:1659-63.

43. Katus HA, Kübler W. Detection of myocardial cell damage in patients with unstable angina by serodiagnostic tools. In: Bleifeld W, Hamm CW, Braunwald E, eds. Unstable angina. Berlin-Heidelberg, Germany: Springer-Verlag, 1990:92-100.

44. Johson RA, Palacios IP. Dilated cardiomyopathies of the adult (second of two parts): acute infectious myopericarditis and acute inflammatory myocarditis. New Engl J Med 1982; 307:1119-26.

45. Woodruff JF. Viral myocarditis. A review. Am J Pathol 1980; 101:427-78.

46. Kawai Ch, Matsumori A, Fujiwara H. Myocarditis and dilated cardiomyopathy. Ann Rev Med 1987; 38:221-39.

47. Dec GW, Palacios IF, Fallon JT et al. Active myocarditis in the spectrum of acute dilated cardiomyopathies. Clinical features, histologic correlates and clinical outcome. New Engl J Med 1985; 312:885-90.

48. Maze SS, Adolph RJ. Myocarditis: unressolved issues in diagnosis and treatment. Clin Cardiol 1990; 13:69-79.

49. Billingham M. Acute myocarditis: a diagnostic dilemma. Br Heart J 1987; 58:6-8.

50. Krasna MJ, Flancbaum L. Blunt cardiac trauma: clinical manifestations and management. Semin Thor Cardiovasc Surg 1992; 4:195-202.

51. Tenzer ML. The spectrum of myocardial contusion: a review. J Trauma 1985; 25:620-7.

52. Fabian TC, Mangiante EC, Patterson LR et al. Myocardial contusion in blunt trauma: clinical characteristics, means of diagnosis and implications for patient management. J Trauma 1988; 28:50-7.

53. Rothstein RJ. Myocardial contusion. JAMA 1983; 250:2189-91.

54. Miller FB, Shumate CR, Richardson JP. Myocardial contusion: when can the diagnosis be eliminated? Arch Surg 1989; 124:805-8.

55. Fabian TC, Cicala RS, Croce MA et al. A prospective evaluation

of myocardial contusion: correlation of significant arrhythmias and cardiac output with CPK-MB measurements. J Trauma 1991; 31,653-60.

56. McLean RF, Devitt JH, McLellan BA et al. Significance of myocardial contusion following blunt chest trauma. J Trauma 1992; 33:240-3.

CHAPTER 3

CONVENTIONAL MARKERS:
LIMITATIONS OF ASPARTATE AMINOTRANSFERASE, CREATINE KINASE AND LACTATE DEHYDROGENASE ISOENZYMES

ASPARTATE AMINOTRANSFERASE (AST)

BIOCHEMISTRY

Aspartate aminotransferase (AST) catalyzes the transfer of an amino group from specific amino acids (L-aspartate or L-glutamate) to specific keto acids (α-oxoglutarate or oxaloacetate) in an important pathway of amino acid metabolism.[1]

$$\text{L-aspartate} + \text{alpha-oxoglutarate} \underset{}{\overset{\text{AST}}{\rightleftharpoons}} \text{oxaloacetate} + \text{L-glutamate}$$

The coenzyme for this reaction is pyridoxal-5'-phosphate. In vivo the reaction produces L-glutamate and oxaloacetate to provide nitrogen for the urea cycle. The produced glutamate is deaminated, which results in the formation of ammonia and regeneration of α-oxoglutarate.

Each AST molecule (MW: 93 kDa) is a dimer composed of two identical subunits. Two genetically and immunologically distinct isoenzymes exist, one located in the cytoplasm (c-AST) and the other in the mitochondria (m-AST).

TISSUE DISTRIBUTION OF AST

AST lacks cardiac specificity. High tissue concentrations of this enzyme are found in the heart and skeletal muscle, liver and kidneys. Lower concentrations are found in pancreas, spleen, lung, and erythrocytes. The AST concentration in myocardium is about 150 U/g wet weight.

AST TIME COURSES AFTER ACUTE MYOCARDIAL INFARCTION

After acute myocardial infarction (AMI), AST rises within 6-12 hours after the onset, peaks about 24 hours and returns within the reference range after 3-6 days.[2] On average, a 5-fold relative increase compared with the upper reference limit is found in AMI patients. c-AST rises before m-AST. m-AST may offer some advantages in estimating the extent of myocardial infarction,[3] but the fundamental problem with this enzyme is lack of cardiac specificity.

CLINICAL SIGNIFICANCE OF AST FOR DIAGNOSING
MYOCARDIAL INJURY

Although this enzyme was the first biochemical marker for AMI, today this enzyme has no clinical significance for the laboratory diagnosis of myocardial damage. AST determination for this purpose is useless and wasteful. Apart from patients with AMI, increases in AST are, for example, found in patients with liver and biliary tract disease, various musculoskeletal disorders, acute pancreatitis, rhabdomyolysis, intestinal injury, local irridation, pulmonary infarction, cerebral infarctions and neoplasms, and renal infarction.

LACTATE DEHYDROGENASE (LDH)

BIOCHEMISTRY

LDH catalyzes the reversible oxidation of lactate to pyruvate, which is essential to the proper function of certain tissues. LDH is responsible for the final step in glycogenolysis (Embden-Meyerhof glycolytic pathway). It is present in the cytoplasm of the cell in large quantities in the majority of human tissues.[2]

$$\text{L-lactate} + NAD^+ \overset{\text{LDH}}{\rightleftharpoons} \text{Pyruvate} + NADH + H^+$$

LDH exists as a tetramer with a molecular weight of 135 kDa. It can be separated by routine electrophoresis into five isoenzymes. Each isoenzyme has been numbered according to its electrophoretic mobility. The fastest migrating fraction (most anodal) is designated LDH-1, the slowest fraction (most cathodic) is LDH-5. LDH is composed of two different subunits, M (muscle; MW approximately 34 kDa) and H (heart; MW approximately 34 kDa). The two subunits are encoded by different genes. It is the combination of these two chains that determines the structure and electrophoretic mobility of each isoenzyme. The polypeptide configuration of each isoenzyme is as follows: LDH-1 (4H), LDH-2 (3HM), LDH-3 (2H2M), LDH-4 (H3M), LDH-5 (4M).

All LDH isoenzymes catalyze the same reversible reaction. However, there is a difference among the isoenzymes as to substrate preference and direction of the reaction.[2,3] Tissues engaged primarily in aerobic metabolism contain more H than M chains and prefer the lactate to pyruvate reaction while tissues more involved in anaerobic metabolism have more M chains and favor the pyruvate to lactate reaction. Thus, the tissue distribution of LDH isoenzymes and their kinetic properties reflect the metabolic requirements. LDH-1 is highly active at low pyruvate concentrations and is inhibited by high pyruvate concentrations. In the heart carbohydrate and fatty acid metabolism is relatively constant and metabolites (e.g., pyruvate) are completely oxidized and LDH-1 is predominant (35-70% of total LDH activity). There are usually no sudden large variations in energy consumption. However, in diseased myocardium (e.g., coronary artery disease and ventricular hypertrophy) the expression of LDH isoenzymes with high M subunit content is enhanced.[3] LDH-5, by contrast, is not inhibited by high pyruvate, and it is less active at low pyruvate concentrations. Fast-twitch skeletal muscle is subject to sudden bursts in activity in which the anaerobic pathways are used for immediate energy requirements. The expression of the M subunit is an adaptation to enhanced use of anaerobic glycogenolysis for energy supply. This may also be the explanation why chronically stressed skeletal muscle (chronic muscle disease, recurrent skeletal muscle injury) reexpresses LDH-1 and LDH-2.[4] In this context it is of interest that slow-twitch skeletal muscle fibers which show a relatively constant state of tonic activity have an LDH isoenzyme pattern similar to that of myocardium.[3]

Tissue Distribution of LDH Isoenzymes

LDH is found in virtually every human tissue with the liver (150-200 U/g), skeletal muscles (150-200 U/g) and the heart (130-170 U/g) having the highest concentrations (in U/g wet weight). The red blood cells (36 U/g hemoglobin), the kidney, the lung, the pancreas and the brain all have about equal amounts of LDH (50-100 U/g).[3,5] Tissue LDH concentrations are mostly about 500-fold higher than serum concentrations. Most tissues contain all isoenzyme types, but LDH-1 and, to a lesser extend, LDH-2 predominate in the heart. LDH-1 is abundant in the myocardium and appears in blood following myocardial damage. But LDH-1 is also predominantly found in brain and also occurs in erythrocytes, pancreas, kidney, stomach, and slow-twitch skeletal muscle fibers. Skeletal muscle and the liver contain mainly LDH-5. The other isoenzymes LDH-2, LDH-3, LDH-4 are found to varying degrees with LDH-1 and LDH-5 in all tissues.

LDH Time Courses After Myocardial Infarction

The rise of total LDH in serum begins 6-12 hours after myocardial damage (see Fig. 3.1). A flipped LDH-1/LDH-2 ratio may be found before total LDH is increased above the upper reference limit. LDH-1 exceeds 50-60% of total LDH activity. LDH peaks at 1-3 days, and returns to baseline 8-14 days after the onset of clinical symptoms. Peak concentrations in AMI patients are about 10-fold the upper reference limit. The reason for the prolonged increase in LDH after AMI is the long biological half-life time of LDH-1 (4-5 days). Clearance of LDH is via the reticuloendothelial system and metabolically highly active tissues (e.g., liver, pancreas, kidneys).[2,3,6-8]

Methods of Determination

Total LDH

Total LDH is measured as enzymatic activity by standardized kinetic assays. Most assays are based on the in vivo reaction (see above), the interconversion of NAD^+ to NADH can be measured spectrophotometrically as absorption at 340 nm. In general, the pyruvate-lactate direction is used because it gives the fastest reaction speed. The presence of macroenzymes of LDH which are prob-

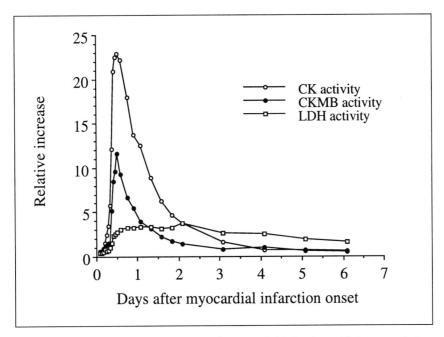

Fig. 3.1. Patient with Q wave anterior wall myocardial infarction with late reperfusion. Concentration time courses are given as relative increases compared with the upper reference limit of enzyme activities (y-axis: 1 represents the upper reference limit). Abbreviations: creatine kinase (CK), lactate dehydrogenase (LDH).

ably complexes of LDH with IgG or IgA lead to false positive increases in total LDH activity.[6,9]

Electrophoresis

Differences in electrophoretic mobility at pH 8.8 on cellulose acetate make it possible to separate the five isoenzymes. LDH-1 is the most rapid (anodic migration) and LDH-5 the slowest. The isoenzymes are visualized by incubation with tetrazolium salt, the intensities of which are measured using densitometry. The value of electrophoresis lies in its ability to discriminate the concentrations of various isoenzymes. Thereby it is possible in many cases to determine the organs affected.[6] The normal LDH isoenzyme relationship in terms of relative concentrations is, in descending order, LDH-2, LDH-1, LDH-3, LDH-4, LDH-5. In the setting of AMI the relative concentrations of LDH-1 and LDH-2 "flip" and LDH-1 exceeds LDH-2, which results in a LDH-1/LDH-2 ratio ≥ 1. The sensitivity of a reversed ratio for AMI is approximately 90% depending on the discriminator. Discriminator values of 0.76 or 0.90-0.95 have been proposed by other investigators.[2,6,10]

2-hydroxybutyrate dehydrogenase (HBDH)

Affinities for pyruvate and certain of its analogs vary between isoenzymes. 2-oxobutyrate is much faster catabolized by LDH-1 and LDH-2 to 2-hydroxybutyrate than by LDH-5. The use of this substrate instead of lactate increases the specificity and HBDH activity is more heart-specific than total LDH activity and is a good indicator of cardiac LDH activity.[6] The HBDH activity in myocardium is about 150-200 U/g wet weight.

Other methods for quantifying LDH-1 isoenzyme

HBDH is not entirely specific for LDH-1. Other methods for measuring LDH-1 include ion-exchange chromatography, immunoprecipitation (anti M-subunit antibodies), and chemical assays, which use selective inhibitors of other enzymes (M-subunit).[6,11] The validity of the latter procedure was questioned.[12] The most promising methods are sensitive and specific immunoassays for LDH-1.[13]

CLINICAL SIGNIFICANCE

Normal human serum contains a considerable amount of circulating LDH due to normal tissue breakdown. LDH-1 does not exceed 40% of total LDH activity. LDH increases above its upper reference limit too late after AMI to be of clinical relevance for triage decisions. But measurement of LDH and the isoenzymes LDH-1 and LDH-2 were widely used for the late diagnosis of myocardial infarction. If the ratio of LDH-1/LDH-2 is >1 myocardial damage is likely and in the absence of hemolysis increases in the LDH-1/LDH-2 ratio and in HBDH are rather specific for myocardial damage. However, erythrocytes, kidneys, brain, pancreas and stomach are other important sources of LDH-1, so that an abnormal serum concentration of LDH-1 may result from irreversible damage to any of these tissues as well. In addition, false positive results were reported in healthy, well-trained athletes and in patients with hemolytic, pernicious, and megaloblastic anemia, intravascular hemolysis, renal ischemia and infarction, muscular dystrophy, and certain tumors of testes and ovaries (seminomas, dysgerminomas). Thus, LDH-1 cannot be regarded as absolutely heart specific. LDH and isoenzymes are less specific than CK and CKMB determinations and add little to the in vitro diagnosis of myocardial damage when CK/CKMB are already diagnostically useful.[14]

However, LDH isoenzymes and HBDH may remain of clinical significance for the noninvasive estimation of myocardial infarction size, because good correlations have been reported with anatomic estimates of infarct size. Due to the very slow elimination of LDH-1 (and HBDH) this marker seems to be superior to CKMB in the estimation of infarct size in patients with reperfusion therapy. Although reperfusion also causes earlier LDH release (see Fig. 3.2), infarct size can be calculated more accurately from the slowly catabolized LDH-1, because a single measurement after 6-8 hours represents approximately the total LDH-1 release over that period and errors are smaller.[15]

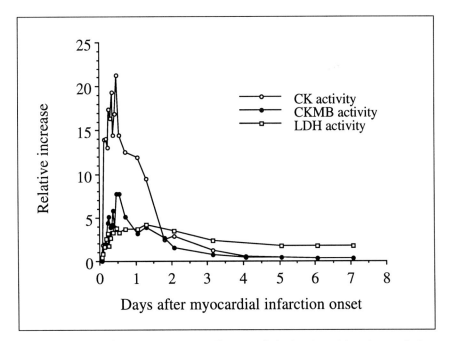

Fig. 3.2. Patient with Q wave anterior wall myocardial infarction with early reperfusion. Concentration time courses are given as relative increases compared with the upper reference limit of enzyme activities (y-axis: 1 represents the upper reference limit). Abbreviations: creatine kinase (CK), lactate dehydrogenase (LDH).

CREATINE KINASE (CK)

BIOCHEMISTRY OF CK

The role of CK in muscle metabolism

CK (molecular weight of about 86 kDa) is an ubiquitious enzyme that functions mainly as a temporal energy buffer and in the transfer of energy from the mitochondria to the cytosol. It is a key enzyme in cellular energetics and in muscular metabolism.[16,17] It is compartmentalized specifically at those places where energy is "produced" or "utilized" (e.g., mitochondria, myofibrils, plasma membrane, sarcoplasmic reticulum). There are two forms, cytosolic and mitochondrial CK. Cytosolic CK shows significant binding to myofibrils (5-10% of cytosolic CK are localized at the M-band). The enzyme can constitute up to 20% of the soluble sarcoplasmic protein in some types of muscle. The majority of studies involving animal hearts or specimens obtained at autopsy from human hearts suggest a uniform distribution of CK and CKMB in normal hearts. CK catalyzes the reversible transfer of a phosphate residue in high energy binding between adenosine triphosphate (ATP) and creatine.

$$\text{Creatine} + \text{ATP} \underset{}{\overset{\text{CK}}{\rightleftharpoons}} \text{Creatine-phosphate} + \text{ADP}$$

The reaction product, creatine phosphate (CP), represents an essential energy store for contraction, relaxation, and transport of substances within the muscle cell. In skeletal muscle CP concentrations may reach 20-35 mM or more.[16] The primary energy source is ATP. In periods of increased demands, however, ATP can be recharged from oxydative phosphorylation and also from CP by CK. The ATP regeneration capacity of CK is high and exceeds both ATP utilization as well as ATP replenishment by oxidative phosphorylation and glycolysis. Thus, CP prevents ATP depletion during the first 4-5 seconds of vigorous exercise while increases in glycolysis and in oxidative phosphorylation are occurring. CK keeps the cellular ADP levels low and prevents the inactivation of ATPases by rising ADP. It also prevents the net loss of cellular adenine nucleotides. Another important function of the CK/CP system is proton buffering, which prevents local or global acidification caused by high ATP breakdown. This is important in the early phase of severe exercise before glycogenolysis is activated. Release of inorganic phosphate from the CK/CP system stimulates indirectly glycogenolysis and glycolysis. Furthermore, CK is also involved in the oxidative phosphorylation in mitochondria of muscle, heart, and brain (mitochondrial CK). Mitochondrial CK acts as an energy conduit from the mitochondrium to the cytoplasma (phosphocreatine circuit).[16] In this role, CP would serve as an "energy carrier" connecting sites of energy production with sites of energy utilization. ATP is generated in the mitochondria and transported through the inner mitochondrial membrane by the adenine nucleotide translocator. Then the mitochondrial CK which is bound to the outer side of the inner mitochondrial membrane catalyzes the phosphorylation of creatine. CP is transferred by facilitated diffusion through the outer mitochondrial membrane into the cytoplasm. The cytosolic CP pool forms an energy store near the sites of energy utilization in the target organelles of the cells, such as myofibrils, plasma membranes and sarcoplasmic reticulum. ATP can be regenerated by the action of CK. Therefore, both ends of the creatine-phosphate shuttle are under control of CK. However, there are probably parallel pathways for ATP and ADP.[16]

To sum up, depending on the metabolic needs of tissues one of these different functions may be dominating. The "energy buffering" function is more prominent in glycolytic, fast-twitch skeletal muscle fibers, which have high levels of cytosolic CK and large CP pools and in which glycolysis is the main pathway of ATP production, the "energy transport" function is more pronounced in oxidative slow-twitch and cardiac muscle, where ATP is mainly derived from fatty acid oxidation within mitochondria. Both muscle types contain relatively high amounts of mitochondrial CK (approximately 15% of total CK).[16]

Molecular forms of CK

Cytosolic CK is a dimeric molecule which is composed of either B subunits (B = brain form; MW 44.5 kDa) or M subunits (M = muscle form; MW 43 kDa). Both subunits are encoded by different genes, thereby providing CK with a certain amount of tissue specificity.[2] Three isoenzymes of cytosolic CK exist; CKBB (CK-1), CKMB (CK-2), and CKMM (CK-3). In addition to the cytosolic forms of CK, there is a mitochondrial form of the enzyme, which is also a dimer and probably consists of two identical subunits (CK-Mi).[18]

Macromolecular forms are occasionally seen in plasma.[19] Macro CK type I (prevalence about 0.5%) is an enzyme-immunoglobulin complex, usually CKBB-IgG. Macro CK type II (prevalence about 1%) is an oligomeric form of mitochondrial CK and probably represents a fragment of the inner mitochondrial membrane. Macro CKs lead to false positive test results in CK activity assays (especially macro CK type I) and in some CKMB assays as well. The presence of macro CK type I is frequently associated with an autoimmune process (especially myositis) and the presence of type II with malignant cell proliferation or severe liver damage (e.g., cirrhosis), respectively.[19] In children macro CK type II is often found with myocardial diseases.[20]

Tissue distribution of CK and its isoenzymes

CK is widely distributed throughout the human body, but it is particularly concentrated in muscle tissue. Clinically significant amounts of total organ activity are found only in skeletal muscle, heart, brain, gut, and pregnant uterus (see Table 3.1), the highest concentration being found in skeletal muscle. All other organs have either insufficient tissue concentration or mass to contribute significantly to serum levels.[21]

CKBB accounts for 100% of the CK in brain. CKBB released from brain can be only detected in the general circulation if the blood-brain barrier is disturbed (e.g., after stroke or trauma).

Depending on sampling site and underlying diseases 3-20% of the total CK activity in myocardial tissue is from CKMB, the remaining percentage being CKMM isoenzyme.[22] The CK activity of myocardium is only about 20-50% of skeletal muscle. The CKMB content of normal myocardium does not differ from skeletal muscle.[22] Recent reports suggest that chronic stress of the myocardium (e.g., ventricular hypertrophy, coronary artery disease) induces the synthesis of CK-B and thus increases the CKMB content of myocardium.[22,23] The rationale of this adaptation process could be the fact that CK-B, as compared with CK-M, favors CP breakdown to ATP especially at low CP levels, whereas CK-M, as compared with CK-B, can catalyze more easily the CP formation process favoring cytoplasmic energy storage.[23] When muscle tissue becomes chronically stressed CP levels could be expected to be

Table 3.1. Tissue distribution of creatine kinase isoenzymes

Tissue	CK activity (U/g wet weight, 30°C)	CKMM (%)	CKMB (%)	CKBB (%)
Skeletal muscle	2500-3000			
fast-twitch (white) fibers		97-99	1-3	<0.1
slow-twitch (red) fibers		90-95	5-10	
Myocardium	500-700			
normal		95	5	
diseased		70-80	20-30	
Brain	200-300			100
Gastrointestinal tract	120-150	<5	<5	>90-95
Bladder	85			100
Uterus				
nonpregnant	165			100
pregnant	245		6	94
Placenta	250	19	1	80
Prostate	85			100
Lung	15	0-20		80-100

chronically decreased. To liberate energy from CP in such situations a high CK-B activity might be necessary.

CKMM accounts for almost all of the CK activity in skeletal muscle. The CKMB content of skeletal muscle varies depending on the proportion of slow-twitch red fibers. The latter may contain up to 5-10% CKMB, whereas fast-twitch white fibers contain about 1-3% or less.[24] Apple et al have demonstrated a correlation between slow-twitch fiber content and CKMB content in gastrocnemius biopsies of long distance runners.[25] With endurance training CKMB accumulates in skeletal muscle and may reach myocardial levels in heart disease.[25] Chronic degeneration and regeneration of skeletal muscle leads to a marked increase in CKMB content. In chronic muscle injury, such as Duchenne muscular dystrophy, the CKMB content of skeletal muscle may reach up to 10-50% of total CK activity.[26] When skeletal muscle is injured, it produces increased amounts of CK-B subunits, just as it does during fetal development.

For all other tissues CKBB accounts for all or most of the CK activity present.[24] These organs contain relatively small CK activity. Because CKBB is cleared rapidly, it is usually only detectable in patients with disease processes that result in continuing release from a tissue with considerable CK content.

Elimination of CK and CKMB from blood

CKMB concentrations found in healthy subjects are low. Skeletal muscle accounts for nearly all the CK including CKMB released into serum, because skeletal muscle has 100 times the mass of myocardium and 5 times its concentration of CK.[17] The enzyme is cleared from the blood by degradation mainly by the liver and other metabolically highly active organs or the reticuloendothelial system.[17] Enzyme elimination generally follows first-order kinetics, the rate of clearance being proportional to the plasma concentration.[27] The biological half-life times of CKMB and CK are about 12-18 hours.

METHODS OF DETERMINATION

Total CK

Assays for CK and CKMB have been extensively reviewed elsewhere.[2,17,28,29] Total serum CK is determined after N-acetylcysteine reactivation of CK by using the hexokinase and glucose-6-phosphate dehydrogenase reaction coupled to the production of ATP and NADPH (monitored by increase in absorbance at 340 nm).[2] Commercial kits contain reagents (e.g., diadenosine pentaphosphate) to inhibit adenylate kinase.[28] This reduces false positive results due to adenylate kinase activity in the sample.

CKMB

CKMB can be detected by a variety of analytical methods[2,6,28,29] that are based on charge differences or on immunological reactivity. Most of these methods cannot be used in the emergency laboratory because they are either time-consuming procedures or not suited for automation. CKMB activity assays do not directly measure the level of the enzyme itself but provide an estimate of CKMB concentration (in standardized international units per liter) based on the enzyme's activity.

Electrophoresis

Electrophoretic separation of CK isoenzymes on agarose gel (or cellulose acetate) followed by their identification by catalytic activity is a commonly used very specific procedure (the visualization is usually based on fluorescence of NADPH produced by the CK-hexokinase-glucose-6-phosphate-dehydrogenase reaction). Sensitivity, however, is limited. The significance of electrophoresis is to identify CK-variants or CKBB. The technique is semiquantitative.

Ion-exchange chromatography for separation of CK isoenzymes

Ion exchange separation of CK isoenzymes on either columns (on DEAE-sepharose A-50 or DEAE-cellulose) or glass beads followed by catalytic CK measurement is also not suited for use in the emergency laboratory because of drawbacks, such as long turn-around time, limited sensitivity, and multiple interferences with the test.[29] Disadvantages of such procedures include dilution of the sample, carry-over of CKMM and Macro CK into the CKMB fraction, little differentiation between CKMB and CKBB and a rather poor precision.[28] This method is not very frequently used.

Immunoinhibition and
immunoinhibition-immunoprecipitation assays

The major types of immunological methods for the determination of CKMB activity are immunoinhibition and immuno-inhibition-immunoprecipitation. Immunoinhibition assays have been widely used in emergency laboratories, because they are easy to handle, ideally suited for automation, sensitive, and provide results rapidly.[30] However any positive result requires confirmation by a more specific method. After addition of anti-M antibodies to inhibit the M-subunit, the residual CK-B activity (non CK-M activity) is quantified spectrophotometrically by measurements of substrate conversion. By multiplication with the factor 2 CKMB activity is calculated. Besides the B-subunit of CKMB, the assay also measures macro CKs, CKBB, and high adenylate kinase activities in serum.

Attempts to improve the specificity of immunoinhibition resulted in the addition of an immunoprecipitation step to remove all M-subunit containing enzymes in a second reaction tube by using specific anti-M antibodies. However, interferences by high

CKBB or CKMM concentrations are still a concern and the immunoinhibition method loses its simplicity and turnaround time becomes longer.

Immunoenzymometric assays (CKMB mass assays)

In contrast with immunoprecipitation and immunoinhibition methods, which measure the isoenzymes by their activity, these immunoassays determine enzyme mass, whether or not the enzyme molecule is catalytically active. Therefore, the presence of endogenous inhibitors and inactivators is not a matter of concern. The introduction of immunoenzymometric CKMB mass assays has improved both the analytical sensitivity and specificity. The latter is due to the fact that CKMM, CKBB, Macro CK Type I and II, and even very high adenylate kinase do not interfere with these assays.[29] These assays have become the method of choice for measurement of CKMB and substantially improved the diagnostic sensitivity of CKMB in clinical practice as well (see chapter 5). The present generation of CKMB immunoassays fulfills the clinical needs for "stat" results.

CK AND CKMB ACTIVITY TIME COURSES AFTER MYOCARDIAL INFARCTION

Following myocardial injury, blood levels of total CK and CKMB activity begin to rise within 4-8 hours. Peak values occur within 24 hours of the onset of AMI and total CK usually returns to baseline within 2-3 days.[2] CKMB peaks slightly earlier and CKMB activity disappears somewhat more rapidly than CK. Recanalization increases the rapidity of the appearance of CK and CKMB in plasma after AMI and peak values occur earlier (see Figs. 3.1 and 3.2). In such cases CKMB may return to normal concentrations within 24 hours. An increase may be found within 2 hours after successful coronary reperfusion and enables earlier confirmation of AMI diagnosis and the detection of failure of recanalization.[31,32]

OTHER SETTINGS

CKMB is not elevated after uncomplicated cardiac catheterization. Patients with increases in CKMB after successful percutaneous transluminal coronary angioplasty are significantly more likely to have had chest pain or small-vessel occlusion during the procedure.[33] These increases do not affect the prognosis of patients. Rhythm disorders do not elevate CKMB. Repetitive, intense countershocks can sometimes lead to increases in CKMB of patients.[2] Closed chest cardiac massage alone usually does not cause an increase in CKMB. Small increases in CKMB may be found in patients with heart failure which may be interpreted as an expression of hypertrophy as well as of degenerative mechanisms. In most patients myocarditis causes detectable CKMB release from the heart.[2] Depending on the methology different percentages of increases in CKMB in patients with unstable angina have been reported.

PITFALLS OF CKMB IN THE DIAGNOSIS OF MYOCARDIAL MUSCLE INJURY

While methodological interferences rarely lead to false positive results using immunoenzymometric CKMB mass assays, CKMB not of myocardial origin can be found in the serum of certain subgroups of patients (see Table 3.2), which may be misleading.[2,6,8,17,25-27] For example, sufficient CKMB can be released from damaged skeletal muscle to increase circulating levels.

The use of a CKMB/total CK index can give improved specificity in patients with concomitant skeletal muscle damage but also leads to an unacceptable loss of sensitivity. The best index value used as a discriminator value for the diagnosis of myocardial damage using a CKMB mass/CK index must be determined in each laboratory, because differences in measuring temperature of CK activity and differences in type and concentrations of activators used in each commercial CK activity assay will alter the decision limit. In patients who sustain an elevation of CKMB based on myocardial injury, the CKMB activity to total CK index usually exceeds 5% and the CKMB mass to CK index exceeds 2.5%, respectively. A major problem is found in cases of simultaneous heart and skeletal muscle injury with CKMB (absolute value or CKMB/CK index). The greater the extent of muscle injury, the more likely that changes in CKMB due to cardiac injury will be missed as CKMB of cardiac origin is "masked" by large quantities of CKMM which decrease the percentage of CKMB. On the other hand, abnormally high relative indices in patients with normal total CK may not be valid indicators. If the serum level of total CK is within normal range, physicians cannot and should not draw any firm

Table 3.2. Common causes of increased serum CKMB in the absence of myocardial damage

1. CKMB release from skeletal muscle
   Trauma
   > "crush injury"
   > burns
   > electrical injuries
   > surgery
   > extreme or unaccustomed exercise

   Grand mal seizures

   Rhabdomyolysis

   Various inflammatory and noninflammatory myopathies
   > polymyositis, dermatomyositis
   > chronic renal failure
   > hypothyroidism
   > chronic alcoholism (especially in delirium tremens and acute alcohol withdrawal)

   Hypo- und hyperthermia

   Resuscitation

   Electric countershock or electroconvulsive therapy

   Poisoning

2. CKMB release from uterus in peripartum period

3. Ektopic CKMB production in tumor patients
   e.g. thyroid and prostatic cancer

4. Decreased clearance from blood
   Hypothyroidism

For methodological reasons of false positive test results see text.

conclusions from the index as to whether patients have myocardial damage. In addition, false positive CKMB results have been reported in patients with renal failure.[2]

Clinical Significance of CKMB

Currently the in vitro diagnosis of myocardial damage is mainly based on the measurement of CKMB. CKMB measurements are widely accepted as an excellent tool for diagnosis of myocardial damage in most patients and, therefore, CKMB has become a cornerstone of diagnosing AMI. In the last quarter century serum levels of CKMB have become the final arbiters by which myocardial damage is diagnosed or excluded. Myocardial cell death of any cause will result in a rising and falling pattern of CKMB (e.g., heart contusion, electrical injury, myocarditis, infarction). Patterns and times of sampling are critical to obtaining results that have meaning. For example, in the case that the patient's hospitalization is very early or delayed after myocardial damage, CKMB levels may be in the normal range. A single set of CK and CKMB activity in the emergency room is not sufficiently sensitive to exclude myocardial infarction, although a single positive result will greatly increase the probability of AMI.[2] In contrast, serial determinations over time have a sensitivity of nearly 100% for detecting AMI.[2] CKMB should be at least measured on admission and about 12 and 24 hours later. Infarct size may be estimated by CKMB measurements, if the amount of enzyme lost from the myocardium, its volume of distribution, and its release ratio are known. The sampling needs to be frequent (at least every 4 hours). However, since the release characteristics are altered by reperfusion, the interpretation becomes much more complex and the perfusion status of the infarct related coronary artery has to be considered. Close correlations of CKMB with other methods to measure infarct size can only be expected in homogenous populations without concomitant skeletal muscle damage with either an early reperfused or closed infarct-related coronary artery. In addition the CKMB content of myocardium may vary within subjects depending on preexisting myocardial diseases (see above). Therefore CKMB seems to be less suitable than cardiac LDH isoenzymes for estimating infarct-size in patients with reperfusion therapy without early angiographically documented success (see above).

In summary, despite the presence of many potential markers, only CK, LDH and their isoenzymes have gained widespread clinical use. However, both markers have drawbacks both in sensitivity and specificity.

REFERENCES
  1. Moss DW, Henderson AR. Enzymes. In: Burtis CA, Ashwood ER, eds. The Tietz Textbook of Clinical Chemistry. 2nd ed. Philadelphia: W.B. Saunders, 1994:788-97.
  2. Lee Th, Goldman L. Serum enzyme assays in the diagnosis of acute myocardial infarction: recommendations based on a quantitative

analysis. Ann Intern Med 1986; 105:221-33.

3. Smith AF, Wilkinson JH. Tissue isoenzymes. In: Hearse DJ, Leiris J Loisance D, eds. Enzymes in Cardiology—Diagnosis and Research. Chichester: J Wiley & Sons, 1979:133-44.

4. Emery AEH. Electrophoretic pattern of lactic dehydrogenase in carriers and patients with Duchenne muscular dystrophy. Nature 1964; 201:1044-5.

5. Wolf PL. Lactate dehydrogenase isoenzymes in myocardial disease. Clin Lab Med 1989; 9:655-65.

6. Smith AF. Enzymes and routine diagnosis. In: Hearse DJ, Leiris J, Loisance D, eds. Enzymes in Cardiology—Diagnosis and Research. Chichester: J Wiley & Sons, 1979:199-246.

7. Friedel R, Diederichs F, Lindena J. Release and extracellular turnover of cellular enzymes. In: Schmidt E, Schmidt FW, Trautschold I, Friedel R, eds. Advances in clinical enzymology. Basel: S. Karger, 1979:70-105.

8. Kupper W, Bleifeld W. Serum enzyme changes in patients with cardiac disease. In: Schmidt E, Schmidt FW, Trautschold I, Friedel R, eds. Advances in clinical enzymology. Basel: S. Karger, 1979:106-23.

9. Harff GA, Backer ET. Radial immunodiffusion and immunoelectrophoresis compared for identifying autoantibodies to lactate dehydrogenase in human serum. Clin Chim Acta 1990; 193:157-64.

10. Jablonsky G, Leung FY, Henderson AR. Changes in the ratio of lactate dehydrogenase isoenzymes 1 and 2 during the first day after acute myocardial infarction. Clin Chem 1985; 31:1621-4.

11. Onigbinde TA, Wu AHB, Johnson M et al. Clinical evaluation of an automated chemical inhibition assay for lactate dehydrogenase isoenzyme 1. Clin Chem 1990; 36:1819-20.

12. Sanders GTP, van der Neut E, van Stralen JP. Inhibition of lactate dehydrogenase isoenzymes by sodium perchlorate evaluated. Clin Chem 1990; 36:1964-6.

13. Liu F, Belding R, Usategui-Gomez M et al. Immunochemical determination of LDH-1. Am J Clin Pathol 1981; 75:701-7.

14. Ellis AK. Serum protein measurements and the diagnosis of acute myocardial infarction (Editorial comment). Circulation 1991; 83:1107-8.

15. de Boer MJ, Suryapranata H, Hoorntje JCA et al. Limitation of infarct size and preservation of left ventricular function after primary coronary angioplasty compared with intravenous streptokinase in acute myocardial infarction. Circulation 1994; 90:753-61.

16. Wallimann T, Wyss M, Brdiczka D et al. Intracellular compartmentation, structure and function of creatine kinase isoenzymes in tissues with high and fluctuating energy demands: the "phosphocreatine circuit" for cellular energy homeostasis (review). Biochem J 1992; 281:21-40.

17. Jones MG, Swaminathan R. The clinical biochemistry of creatine kinase. J Int Fed Clin Chem 1990; 2:108-14.

18. Payne RM, Haas RC, Strauss A. Structural characterization and tissue-specific expression of the mRNAs encoding isoenzymes from two rat mitochondrial creatine kinase genes. Biochim Biophys Acta 1991; 1089:352-61.

19. Lee KN, Csako G, Bernhardt P et al. Relevance of macro creatine kinase type 1 and 2 isoenzymes to laboratory and clinical data. Clin Chem 1994; 40:1278-83.

20. Wu AHB, Herson VC, Bowers GN Jr. Macro creatine kinase types 1 and 2: clinical significance in neonates and children as compared with adults. Clin Chem 1983; 29:201-4.

21. Neumaier D. Tissue specific distribution of creatine kinase isoenzymes. In: Lang H, ed. Creatine kinase isoenzmes—pathophysiology and clinical application. Berlin-Heidelberg-New York: Springer-Verlag, 1981:31-83.

22. Ingwall JS, Kramer MF, Fifer MA et al. The creatine kinase system in normal and diseased human myocardium. New Engl J Med 1985; 313:1050-4.

23. Sylven C, Lin L, Kallner A et al. Dynamics of creatine kinase shuttle enzymes in the human heart. Eur J Clin Invest 1991; 21:350-4.

24. Lott JA, Wolf PL. Clinical enzymology. New York: Field, Rich & Associates Inc, 1986:164-7.

25. Apple FS, Rogers MA, Sherman WM et al. Profile of creatine kinase isoenzymes in skeletal muscle of marathon runners. Clin Chem 1984; 30:413-6.

26. Somer H, Duboeitz V, Donner M. Creatine kinase isoenzymes in neuromuscular diseases. J Neurol Sci 1976; 29:129-36.

27. Roberts R, Sobel BE. The distribution, inactivation and clearance of enzymes. In: Hearse DJ, Leiris J, Loisance D, eds. Enzymes in Cardiology—Diagnosis and Research. Chichester: J Wiley & Sons, 1979:97-114.

28. Helger R, Hennich N, Würzburg U et al. Methods for differentiation and quantitation of creatine kinase isoenzymes. In: Lang H, ed. Creatine kinase isoenzmes—pathophysiology and clinical application. Berlin-Heidelberg-New York: Springer-Verlag, 1981:31-83.

29. Chan KM, Ladenson JH, Pierce GF et al. Increased creatine kinase in the absence of acute myocardial infarction (Washington University Case Conference). Clin Chem 1986; 32:2044-51.

30. Obzansky D, Lott JA. Clinical evaluation of an immunoinhibition procedure for creatine kinase MB. Clin Chem 1980; 26:150-2.

31. Garabedian HD, Gold HK, Yasuda T et al. Detection of coronary artery reperfusion with creatine kinase-MB determination during thrombolytic therapy: correlation with acute angiography. J Am Coll Cardiol 1988; 11:729-34.

32. Grande P, Granborg J, Clemmensen P et al. Indices of reperfusion

in patients with acute myocardial infarction using characteristics of the CKMB time-activity curve. Am Heart J 1991; 122:400-8.

33. Oh JK, Shub C, Ilstrup DM et al. Creatine kinase release after successful percutaneous transluminal coronary angioplasty. Am Heart J 1985; 109:1225-31.

CHAPTER 4

FEATURES OF AN IDEAL MARKER

As outlined in detail in the previous chapter, increases in CK and LDH isoenzymes are not as sensitive and heart-specific as first believed, which initiated the search for alternative, possibly more sensitive and specific parameters. Thus, what are the features of the ideal marker we are looking for?

To meet the clinical requirements (see chapter 2) a marker must fulfill several demands (see Table 4.1). An ideal myocardial marker should allow to discriminate between irreversible myocardial damage and reversible minimal changes. This means that the marker should either increase only after irreversible myocardial necrosis or only after reversible myocardial damage. A marker should be absolutely heart-specific to allow reliable diagnosis of myocardial damage in the presence of skeletal muscle injury (e.g., perioperative myocardial infarction, heart contusion). It should be highly sensitive and should detect even small damage (e.g., unstable angina, cardiotoxic or infectious myocarditis). For this purpose it is necessary that a marker is not detectable in patients without myocardial damage and that high amounts are present in cardiomyocytes, which leads to a high serum entry ratio in case of myocardial damage and allows the detection of even small areas of damage. Most of the protein should arrive unaltered in blood. The marker must be suitable for early as well as late diagnosis (broad diagnostic window). Increases should be detectable within 3 hours or earlier after the onset of damage in the majority of patients, and the marker should stay elevated for about a week. This could facilitate early diagnosis of acute myocardial infarction (AMI) in patients with nondiagnostic presenting electrocardiograms. In AMI the marker should allow to monitor reperfusion therapy and to estimate infarct size and prognosis. Of particular interest is to reliably identify patients with failed thrombolytic treatment who may benefit from further interventions (e.g., rescue coronary angioplasty). Consequently, measurement must be rapid (a quantitative whole-blood bedside assay is desirable), easy to perform, quantitative and finally cost effective.

This listing suggests that a single marker can hardly combine all these characteristics and a combination of marker measurement may be necessary. In the next chapter new markers or measuring methods will be introduced and discussed in detail.

Table 4.1. Features of an ideal marker for myocardial damage

- Discrimination between "reversible minimal changes" and irreversible myocardial damage
- Monitoring of thrombolytic therapy in patients with myocardial infarction
- Estimate myocardial infarction size and prognosis
- Absolute cardiac-specificity
- High sensitivity
- High stability
- Early and late diagnosis
- Rapid measurement (whole-blood assay), easy to perform, quantitative, and cost effective

---

CHAPTER 5

NEW MARKERS

PROTEIN CONCENTRATION
OF CREATINE KINASE MB (CKMB MASS)

Although the first radioimmunoassays for measuring CK isoenzymes and specific immunoradiometric assays for CKMB determination were developed around 1980,[1-3] the breakthrough for this new CKMB determination method in routine laboratories took longer. Around 1990 the first rapid immunoenzymometric assays which are performed using fully automated analyzers were available. During recent years CKMB activity assays have been increasingly replaced by CKMB mass assays which measure the protein concentration of CKMB rather than its catalytic activity. Enzymeimmunoassays are presently used in the majority of laboratories throughout the USA and Canada for measurement of CKMB.[4] Rapid quantitative CKMB mass assays are available. The determination is available on many different analytical systems, and results can often be obtained within 15-30 minutes of specimen receipt. These analytical systems are robust so that an available 24-hour service is possible. In addition, a semiquantitative whole blood assay for bedside determination of CKMB mass is available as well. With these immunoassays analytical interferences which lead to false positive test results are also less frequent than with CKMB activity assays[5] (see chapter 3). CKMM, CKBB, macro CKs, and adenylate kinase do not interfere with these immunoassays. Apart from being more specific the quantitative immunoassays also have a higher analytical sensitivity with an improved signal to noise ratio in the low measuring range compared with the currently available activity assays. Enzymeimmunoassays have become the method of choice for measuring CKMB in the routine laboratory. However, a standardization of all commercially available CKMB enzymeimmunoassays is urgently needed and overdue. It can be expected that standardized CKMB mass assays will be soon available, because a suitable reference material (recombinant CKMB) has been found.[6] This will allow to compare the results of studies in which assays of different manufacturers were used for CKMB mass determination.

EARLY SENSITIVITY OF CKMB MASS
FOR ACUTE MYOCARDIAL INFARCTION

The first hints that CKMB mass might be more sensitive for the early diagnosis of AMI were found using the early immunoradiometric assays.[3,7] Later on a concordance between CKMB mass and CKMB activity was frequently reported in the literature.[8] However, in these studies the sampling regimens were not suited to detect the important differences in early sensitivities. Around 1990 the first larger studies were published which clearly demonstrated the higher early sensitivity of CKMB mass and the clinical benefits of CKMB mass determination for medical decision making in triaging chest pain patients.[9-11] Newly improved immunoassays allow physicians to measure CKMB more rapidly and with far greater sensitivity in patients suspect for having an acute myocardial infarction (AMI). After AMI increased CKMB mass concentrations are usually found on average 1 hour earlier than increased CKMB activities in the same patients (see Fig. 5.1). The early sensitivities of CKMB mass and myoglobin are roughly comparable.[12] Abnormal levels of CKMB mass are found within 3 hours from the onset of coronary artery occlusion in up to 50% of patients who develop an AMI, and within 6 hours after symptom onset CKMB mass concentrations are abnormal in approximately 80-100% of patients. Persistently normal CKMB mass concentrations over a period of 6-8 hours have a negative predictive value of about 95%.[13] CKMB mass concentrations stay increased for about 2-3 days. It was also suggested that serial determinations of CKMB mass are diagnostically more effective,[9,14] because a single sampling of CKMB early after the onset of symptoms does not rule out AMI. The importance of CKMB mass determination for rapid diagnosing of AMI in patients with nondiagnostic presenting electrocardiogram (ECG) could be convincingly demonstrated by recent clinical studies.[13-15] Therefore, these assays are today widely used for the early diagnosis of AMI.

CKMB MASS TO MONITOR REPERFUSION IN AMI PATIENTS FOLLOWING SYSTEMIC THROMBOLYTIC TREATMENT

Early detection of failure of recanalization could allow for mechanical intervention or "second shot" thrombolytic therapy to reperfuse ischemic myocardium. After reperfusion, the release ratios of CK and CKMB and their rates of egress into the circulation increase,[16] which aids detection of reperfusion. However, only criteria which are based on the early rate or relative early increase of CKMB are useful to monitor thrombolytic therapy, because only in these circumstances is an early intervention possible if needed. Several criteria have been established in acute coronary angiography controlled studies. A summary is listed in Table 5.1. Criteria based

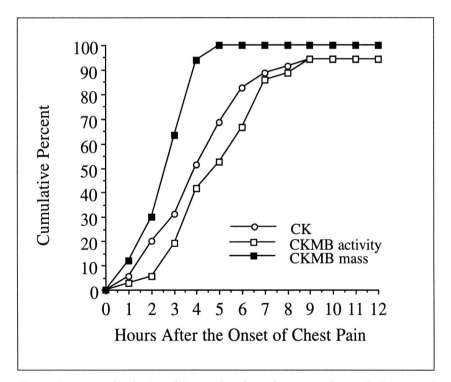

Fig. 5.1. Frequency distribution of times to first above the upper reference limit increased CKMB mass, CKMB and total CK catalytic concentrations of 37 patients with acute myocardial infarction.

Table 5.1. Suggested CKMB mass concentration criteria for the discrimination between myocardial infarction patients with and without reperfusion

Suggested Threshold	Sensitivity	Specificity	Patency defined as
Slope > 17.5 µg/L/h (ref. 17,19)	0.77 – 0.87	0.61 – 0.71	TIMI grade 2 or 3
2.2-fold increase in 90 minutes in inferior AMI* (refs. 18,19)	0.68 – 0.77	0.56 – 1.0	TIMI grade 2 or 3
2.5-fold increase in 90 minutes in anterior AMI* (refs. 18,19)	0.61 – 0.92	0.53 – 1.0	TIMI grade 2 or 3
4-fold increase in 90 minutes* (ref. 19)	0.45 – 0.60	0.68 – 0.81	TIMI grade 3
Slope > 24 µg/L/h (ref. 19)	0.50 – 0.70	0.70	TIMI grade 3

* For example, a 4-fold increase means a 4-fold increase compared to baseline values before start of thrombolytic therapy in a given time period.
   Definition of the perfusion of the infarct-related coronary artery in the Thrombolysis in Myocardial Infarction (TIMI) trial (61):
   Grade 0 = no perfusion; grade 1 = penetration of the contrast material without perfusion; grade 2 = partial perfusion; grade 3 = complete perfusion

on time-to-CKMB peak values are not listed. Such a monitoring can be only used for documentation and has no effects on patient care, because it is simply too late to salvage myocardium.

CKMB MASS IN PATIENTS WITH UNSTABLE ANGINA

Conventional markers are almost always unchanged in unstable angina. Increases in CKMB mass are, however, much more frequently observed than CKMB activity increases in patients with unstable angina. There are two temporal CKMB mass patterns—stable and fluctuating CKMB concentrations (see Fig. 5.2). These patients with increased CKMB mass are a high risk subgroup.[20] Cardiac events are frequent in this subgroup of patients with unstable angina.[21] Even if CKMB mass is only increased between one- and twofold the upper reference limit, this indicates a higher risk of cardiac death, of developing an AMI or requiring revascularization during the subsequent months. Their prognosis

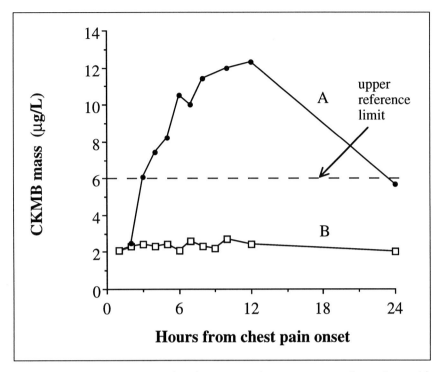

Fig. 5.2. CKMB mass concentration time courses in two representative patients with unstable angina: one with (A) and one without (B) a temporary increase in CKMB mass.

is comparable to patients with a myocardial infarction. CKMB mass assays performed on patients with unstable angina can have an important prognostic function, as they probably indicate the occurrence of ongoing microinfarction.

CKMB MASS CONCENTRATIONS AFTER
INVASIVE CARDIOLOGICAL INTERVENTIONS

These enzymeimmunoassays are capable of detecting even very limited myocardial injury. Thus, increases in CKMB mass may be found after multiple endomyocardial biopsies or following radiofrequency ablation electrical therapy for rhythm disturbances.[22] CKMB mass concentrations are not increased in the systemic circulation after visually successful percutaneous transluminal coronary angioplasty (PTCA), if baseline values were within the reference interval.[23,24] However, CKMB mass is a sensitive marker to detect complications during or after the procedure.[23,24] Moderate increases are found after even minor complications, such as side-branch occlusion (even when symptomless), or severe episodes of myocardial ischemia (see Fig. 5.3). Increases are marked when myocardial infarction occurs (see Fig. 5.3). After PTCA-related procedures, such as directional coronary atherectomy, coronary stenting or coronary rotational ablation slight or moderate increases in CKMB mass concentrations are frequently (in about 10-15% of patients) found even in otherwise uncomplicated patients (see Fig. 5.3). In general, this has no adverse clinical consequences and should not be considered a major complication.

CKMB Mass in the Diagnosis of Perioperative Myocardial Infarctions in Coronary Artery Bypass Grafting

After coronary artery bypass grafting the usual CKMB mass reference limits are invalid as a consequence of inevitable cardiac (cardioplegic cardiac arrest with right atriotomy or intermittent aortic cross clamping) and extracardiac tissue damage occurring during the surgical procedure. However, CKMB release from skeletal muscle is usually small and negligible. The interpretation of CKMB

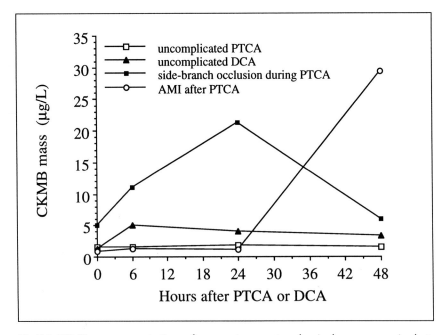

Fig. 5.3. CKMB mass concentrations after percutaneous transluminal coronary angioplasty (PTCA) or directional coronary atherectomy (DCA). Abbreviations: acute myocardial infarction (AMI).

elevation is considerably more complex. Only increases in CKMB of more than 12-18 hours correlate well with other evidence for myocardial infarction.[25] CKMB release is a very valuable routine complementary criterion to an ECG in the diagnosis of perioperative myocardial infarction after coronary bypass surgery.[26] CKMB mass concentrations could better differentiate the patients with AMI from the uncomplicated cases after CABG than all the other CKMB activity measuring methods tested (immunoinhibition, immunoinhibition-immunoprecipitation, column chromatography, electrophoresis).[27] In uncomplicated cases CKMB peak concentrations occur within 6-10 hours from aortic unclamping and do not exceed 75 µg/l.[26] CKMB mass returns to normal within 24-48 hours from aortic unclamping. In patients with myocardial infarction CKMB mass peaks occur between about 16-24 hours after unclamping and a single CKMB mass determination at 12-20 hours after unclamping (discriminator value 50 µg/L) differentiates patients with and without perioperative myocardial infarction (see Fig. 5.4).[28]

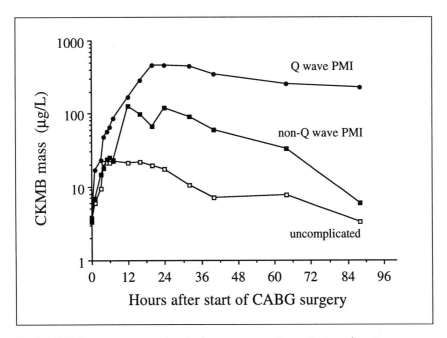

Fig. 5.4. CKMB mass concentrations in three representative patients undergoing coronary artery bypass surgery, one with perioperative Q wave, one with perioperative non-Q wave infarction, and one uncomplicated course. Abbreviations: coronary artery bypass grafting (CABG), perioperative myocardial infarction (PMI).

SPECIFICITY OF CKMB MASS—RELATIVE INDEX OF CKMB MASS OVER TOTAL CK ACTIVITY

Although CKMB mass is more specific than CK, false positive results do occur. Elevations based on noncardiac sources encompass for example trauma, surgery or disease of skeletal muscle, small intestine, uterus, and prostate, as well as patients with rhabdomyolysis, dermatomyositis, polymyositis, Reye's syndrome, hypothyroidism that occurs peripartum, and neoplasms of the lung, breast and kidney (see chapter 3). Distinguishing CKMB elevations due to myocardial injury from those due to skeletal-muscle damage can be difficult. For this purpose it has been frequently recommended to measure CKMB mass as a percentage of total CK activity. This is based on the premise that there is a higher percentage of CKMB in cardiac than in skeletal muscle, which, however, only holds for diseased myocardium (see chapter 3). In addition, high relative indices in patients with normal total CK activity are not reliable indicators and should not be used for medical decision making. The limitations of a CKMB over CK index are discussed in detail in chapter 3. In summary positive CKMB mass values must also be critically analyzed to exclude a noncardiac source of increased values in serum and should never be used as the sole diagnostic indicator. This is particularly important when patients with multiple medical problems with a low to medium probability of myocardial damage are being tested.

CREATINE KINASE ISOFORMS

Another possibility to increase the sensitivity of CKMB isoenzyme is to determine its isoforms in plasma.[29] Unlike atypical CK forms (macro CKs, see chapter 3), which only appear in serum on rare occasions, the CKMB and CKMM isoforms are part of the usual clearance process of the CK isoenzymes and are present in all human sera. Isoenzyme subforms (isoforms) have different isoelectric points, but similar enzymatic activity, and the presence of the isoforms does not appear to affect the determination of total CKMB or CK.

The human myocardium and skeletal muscles contain a single MM and a single MB isoform.[30,31] The native isoforms in myocardium are $CKMB_2$ and $CKMM_3$. After release from the tissue the native isoforms are modified by serum carboxypeptidase N to produce additional CK isoforms.[32] This enzyme cleaves the carboxy terminal lysine from each M subunit,[33] and there are at least two CKMB and three CKMM isoforms. In the serum isoform MM_2 the C-terminal lysine of one M subunit has been cleaved and in the serum isoform MM_1 the lysine residues of both M subunits were cleaved by carboxypeptidase. Both serum isoforms of the MM isoenzyme are produced in a stepwise fashion. The M subunit of the serum isoform of the MB isoenzyme (MB_1) has no C-terminal lysine. Recent studies[34,35] suggest that the native subunit B itself undergoes a structural change through removal of a C-terminal lysine by carboxypeptidase N. CKMB is therefore also constituted of three isoforms, and the CKBB isoenzyme would also consist of three isoforms. However, due to the insufficient resolution of the currently used techniques (high-voltage electrophoresis) for CK isoform determination in routine clinical laboratories, usually only two CKMB and three CKMM isoforms (the five major CK isoforms) are detected, and the CKBB isoenzyme is considered homogeneous.

SEPARATION AND DETERMINATION OF CK ISOFORMS

Electrophoresis

The most frequently applied method for measurement of CK-isoforms in the routine laboratory is high-voltage electrophoresis.[36] A fully automated system with computer-assisted interpretation of the results is commercially available for the rapid isoform determination in the emergency laboratory. After electrophoresis on agarose gels a reagent showing CK activity is applied so that the bands can be visualized using fluorescence or scanned densitometrically. Results are available within 30 minutes. The five main CK isoforms, two MB isoforms and the three conventional MM isoforms, can be separated by this technique. In addition to the three MM isoforms, a fourth subband more anodic than MM_1 can be frequently detected in plasma samples using this technique. In normal plasma only low activities of the MB isoforms are found. The MB_2/MB_1 ratio using this technique is approximately one in healthy individuals.[36] A MB_2 activity of ≥ 1 U/L together with an MB_2/MB_1 ratio ≥ 1.5 indicates myocardial damage. The MM_3/MM_1 ratio in plasma of individuals without muscle damage is always below one, a ratio >0.7 indicates muscle damage.[12,37-39]

Isoelectric focusing

Isoelectric focusing has been the most widely used technique for scientific investigations on CK isoforms in serum and tissues. This method consists of separating native and modified isoforms on the basis of their electric charge. Separation is carried out on thin polyacrylamide or agarose gel slides using ampholytes ranging in pH from 4.5 to 8. The isoelectric points (pI) on agarose slides are about 6.9, 6.7, and 6.2 for MM_3, MM_2, and MM_1, and 5.2 and 5.1 for MB_2 and MB_1, respectively. Isoelectric focusing lasts between 30 and 120 minutes. After separation the gels are incubated with reagents revealing CK activity, and CK bands are visualized similar to electrophoresis by fluorescence under UV light, or scanned densitometrically. Isoelectric focusing is among the techniques with the best resolution of all current methods. Thus, at least one isoform migrating anodic to MM_1 and at least two isoforms migrating cathodic to MM_3 (pI 7.3 and 7.1; MM_4 pI 7.1) and at least one additional MB isoform (MB_3 pI 5.4) have been demonstrated using this method.[35,40] These additional minor MM isoforms are labile intermediates from oxidation or reduction of MM_3 and MM_1, respectively[40] and are clearly mixed with MM_3 and MM_1 by electrophoresis. MB_1 and MB_2 are difficult to separate on electrophoresis, because the difference of pI between MB_2 and MB_1 is only 0.1. In fact the tissue isoform MB_2 of electrophoresis corresponds to MB_3 of isoelectric focusing and the plasma isoform MB_1 of electrophoresis is a mixture of two plasma isoforms MB_2 and MB_1 of isoelectric focusing. In this MB_2 isoform the C-terminal lysine of the B subunit is cleaved, MB_1 has no C-terminal lysines on both the B and the M subunit.[41] The detection of these additional CK isoforms by isoelectric focusing does not seem to improve the diagnostic performance of CK isoforms for the early diagnosis of AMI.[40] Since isoelectric focusing requires time and complicated techniques, the method may not be suitable for routine work.

Chromatofocusing chromatography

This technique is similar in principle to isoelectric focusing, separating isoforms on the basis of their isoelectric points. Samples are injected onto a packed column and are eluted by a pH gradient that is varied. Individual isoforms are collected and assayed for CK activity.[42] The resolution is not as good as that of isoelectric focusing and this method cannot be used in the emergency laboratory either.

High-pressure liquid chromatography (HPLC) and high performance capillary electrophoresis (HPCE)

CK isoenzymes and isoforms can be separated and measured by HPLC on anion-exchange columns[43] and methods based on HPCE are currently being developed. At present these techniques are more research tools.

Immunological methods

The development of immunological techniques for CK isoform determination is hampered by the fact that the major CK isoforms differ only by a single C-terminal amino acid. Consequently it is very difficult to produce specific antibodies.

Immunoinhibition-immunoextraction: Catalytic activities of MM_3 and MB_2 can be measured as the difference between the total CK activity and the activity of the sample after inhibition or removal of the tissue isoform using specific antibodies. One commercially available technique uses antibody-coated paramagnetic particles for the extraction of $CKMM_3$ from the sample. Another assay uses two antibodies for the joint extraction of all MM isoforms and MB_1 isoform, and the activity of residual MB_2 and BB isoenzyme activity is measured. Using an anti M antibody CKMM and CKMB isoenzymes are removed, and the residual BB activity in the sample can be measured. By subtraction it is possible to calculate the MB_2 activity of the sample. Another commercially available immunoinhibition assay for the measurement of native tissue MM and MB isoforms is based on a monoclonal antibody which specifically inhibits the native M subunit of CK.[44] The antibody does not inhibit the M subunit modified by removal of lysine by plasma carboxypeptidase N. This procedure cannot separate tissue MM and MB isoform activity.

The native MB_2 isoform may be also determined as mass concentration. MB mass is determined before and after immunoextraction of the MB_1 isoform by a specific antibody and the difference allows to quantify the mass concentrations of both MB isoforms.

However, all these techniques are either not sufficiently specific or not fully automated and as a consequence not ideal methods for the emergency laboratory. In summary, at present fully automated high-voltage electrophoresis seems to be the most specific, practical and least costly of all introduced methods for the CK isoform determination in routine clinical and emergency analysis.

CK ISOFORM TIME COURSES
AFTER ACUTE MYOCARDIAL INFARCTION

Of the three main MM isoforms MM_3 is the first to rise in the blood after AMI, which is mainly responsible for the increase in total CK activity (see Fig. 5.5). The maximum percentages of MM_3 are recorded 6-12 hours after onset of symptoms.[12,37,38,40,43] In the following hours there is a progressive shift in which MM_3 decreases whereas the transformation products MM_2 and MM_1 increase. Peak activities of MM_3 are found before MM_2 peaks, and MM_1 peaks after MM_2 (see Fig. 5.5). MM_1 becomes the prominent isoform of the MM fraction after approximately 24 hours. The MM_3/MM_1 ratio reaches peak values within 12 hours from the onset of chest pain and then rapidly falls within the reference interval approximately 24 hours after the onset of symptoms. In the very first hours after AMI onset the MB_2 isoform represents in blood usually more than 90% of the total CKMB fraction.[12,29,36-38,40,43] There is than a rapid change in the relative proportions of the two isoforms, with the percentage of MB_2 rapidly dropping during the following hours and MB_1 becomes the predominant isoform after 12-16 hours and the MB isoform ratio returns to normal. The maximum MB_2/MB_1 ratios are found within 8 hours from the onset of symptoms usually before the MM_3/MM_1 ratio peaks.

A flipped tissue to serum isoform ratio is usually found before total CK or CKMB activities increase above their upper reference limits in plasma (see Fig. 5.6).[12,29,37,38,40] However, we and others could demonstrate that the early sensitivity of CKMB isoforms and CKMB are equivalent when sensitive enzymeimmunoassays are used for total CKMB measurement.[12,37] Myoglobin and CK isoform ratios have a comparable early sensitivity.[12,40] Myoglobin, CKMB mass and CK isoforms are, however, considerably more sensitive than CK and CKMB activities[12] (see Figs. 5.6 and 5.7).

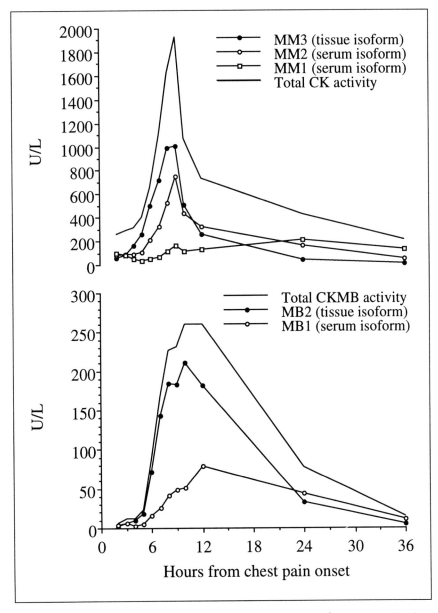

Fig. 5.5. CK isoform time courses in comparison to total CK and CKMB activities in a patient with anterior wall Q-wave myocardial infarction.

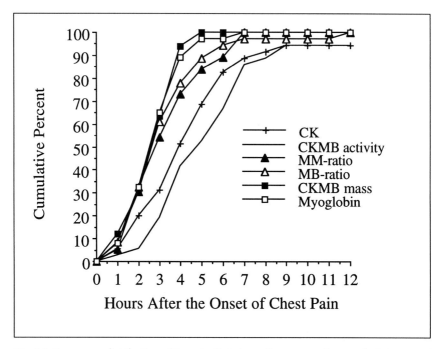

Fig. 5.6. Frequency distribution of times to first above the upper reference limit increased myoglobin, CKMB mass, CKMM and CKMB isoform ratios, and CKMB and total CK activities of 37 patients with acute myocardial infarction.

CK isoforms may also be used as indicators of reperfusion after thrombolytic therapy (see Table 5.2). CKMM and CKMB isoforms are early and sensitive markers of successful thrombolysis.[19,45] CK isoform ratios increase and peak significantly more rapidly in reperfused than in nonreperfused patients (see Fig. 5.8). However, early sampling is essential if additional interventions are to be implemented based on the results and only such criteria are listed in Table 5.2. The largest study so far published on the diagnostic performance of CK isoforms to detect reperfusion[45] could not demonstrate more than limited clinical usefulness. Because of the substantial overlap between patients with and without reperfusion no cut-off values for clinical use are proposed by the authors of this study, although they demonstrated significant differences between both patient groups.

CK ISOFORMS IN OTHER CARDIAC DISEASES

Myocardial injury other than infarction may also be detectable by analysis of CK isoforms. Increases in CKMB isoform ratios were

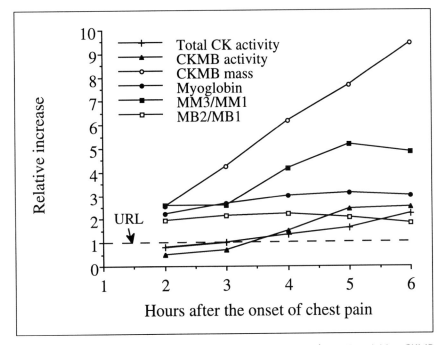

Fig. 5.7. CK isoform ratio time courses in comparison to CK and CKMB activities, CKMB mass, and myoglobin in a patient with anterior wall non-Q wave myocardial infarction. Time courses are given as relative increases compared to the upper reference limit (URL) of each parameter. CK and CKMB activities increased about 1-2 hours later than the other markers which were already increased on admission.

found in patients with less overt damage than myocardial infarction, such as unstable angina, cardiac transplant rejection and cardio-myopathy.[38] Coronary angiography does not lead to change in CK isoform ratios. Patients undergoing PTCA showed an association between ischemic ST segment changes lasting more than 3 minutes (indicating acute coronary ischemia) and a transient increase in the MB isoform ratio, although all patients had total CKMB activity within normal limits. In CABG patients without perioperative myocardial infarction the CKMB isoform ratio mostly peaks about 1 hour after aortic unclamping and returns to baseline by 24 hours after surgery. The CKMM isoform ratio peaks 1-2 hours later.[38]

MM ISOFORMS IN NONMYOCARDIAL DISEASES

Since CKMM isoforms are not specific for myocardium, their utilization for the diagnosis of AMI requires that acute skeletal muscle damage is excluded. On the other hand, CKMM isoforms

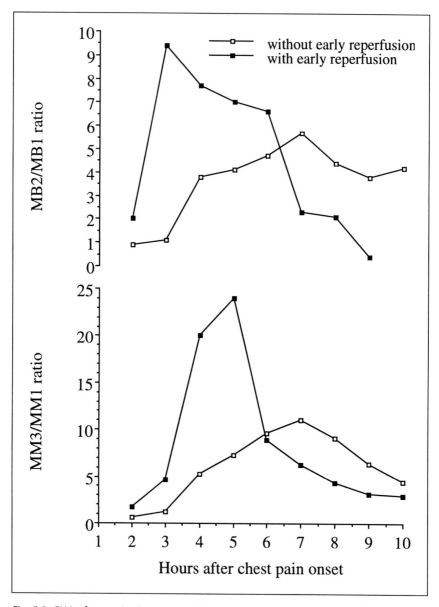

Fig. 5.8. CK isoform ratio time courses in two representative patients with and without early reperfusion of the infarct-related coronary artery. The more rapid increase in isoform ratios in reperfused patients is illustrated.

Table 5.2. Suggested CK isoform criteria for the discrimination between myocardial infarction patients with and without reperfusion

Suggested Threshold	Sensitivity	Specificity	Patency defined as
$CKMM_3$ Slope > 0.2%/min (ref. 19)	0.50 – 0.65	0.65 – 0.85	TIMI grade 3
$CKMM_3/CKMM_1$ Slope > 1%/min (ref. 19)	0.50 – 0.75	0.60 – 0.70	TIMI grade 3
$CKMM_3$ Relative increase >0.4 (ref. 19)*	0.70	0.55 – 0.75	TIMI grade 3
$CKMM_3/CKMM_1$ Relative increase >2* (ref. 19)	0.50 – 0.70	0.60 – 0.90	TIMI grade 3

* For example, a relative increase >2 means a 2-fold increase compared to baseline values before start of thrombolytic therapy in a given time period.
  Definition of the perfusion of the infarct-related coronary artery in the Thrombolysis in Myocardial Infarction (TIMI) trial (61):
  Grade 0 = no perfusion; grade 1 = penetration of the contrast material without perfusion; grade 2 = partial perfusion; grade 3 = complete perfusion

may find an application in patients with skeletal muscle diseases (e.g., polymyositis, Duchenne muscular dystrophy). In patients with chronic stable muscle diseases the MM_1 concentration should be higher than MM_3 although the total CK activity may be increased, because MM_3 has roughly a twofold shorter biological half-life than MM_1.[43,46] Worsening of the disease leads to acute muscle damage and a flipped CKMM isoform ratio. Skeletal muscle trauma and exercise can also cause increased CKMM isoforms with an abnormal ratio in plasma.[43]

CLINICAL SIGNIFICANCE OF CK ISOFORMS

CKMB isoforms are a good test for ruling in and ruling out AMI under the proper clinical conditions, that are the patient must be a chest pain patient and should be hemodynamically stable, and the sample must be drawn within the first 8-10 hours of chest pain onset. As a rule, a rising MB_2 along with an increasing

MB_2/MB_1 ratio indicates a recent myocardial injury within the preceding 2-6 hours. A stagnant MB_2 with a stagnant MB isoform ratio suggests no recent myocardial injury. An MB_2 activity >7 U/L at 6-8 hours after the onset of chest pain indicates AMI with high probability; a patient with <2 U/L at this time has probably no myocardial injury. As with the other markers (myoglobin, CKMB mass) at least three samples (e.g., 3-4 hours, 5-6 hours, 8-10 hours from chest pain onset) should be taken in patients with suspected AMI, and about 10 hours from the onset of the attack have to be awaited before an AMI may be ruled out (cut-off values of MB_2 <2.6 U/L and MB_2/MB_1 ratio <1.7 are recommended when using high-voltage electrophoresis).

For the interpretation of CK isoform results it has to be also taken into account that serum concentrations of carboxypeptidase can vary considerably in patients, which may lead to false positive or negative CK isoform ratios.[47] Carboxypeptidase is synthesized in the liver and secreted into the blood. Enzyme levels are elevated during pregnancy and in patients with certain types of cancer and are low in patients with cirrhosis of the liver. There can be up to a threefold variation among normal persons as well.

The tissue distribution and specificity of CKMM and CKMB isoforms for irreversible injury are the same as those for CK and CKMB. Therefore also other than cardiac sources may lead to an increase in MB_2 activity and MB isoform ratio, for example, extreme exercise, trauma, surgery, polymyositis, dermatomyositis, rhabdomyolysis, delirium tremens, renal failure, thyroid and prostatic cancer, peripartum period, or carbon monoxide poisoning (see chapter 3).

Finally, although CKMB isoform determination is clearly more sensitive than CKMB activity measurements, up to now no significant advantages of CKMB isoform over CKMB mass concentration determination could be demonstrated.

MYOGLOBIN

Myoglobin is an oxygen-binding heme protein of low molecular mass (MW: 17.8 kDa). It is only found in striated muscles, where it accounts for 5-10% of all cytoplasmatic proteins (myoglobin concentration: approximately 4-5 mg/g wet weight). It is not found in smooth muscle. Myoglobin is an oxygen transport protein and is located in the striated muscle fibers close to the sarcolemma, to the contractile apparatus, and to intracellular membranous or fibrillar structures. In skeletal muscle myoglobin is mainly found in the slow-twitch ("red") fibers. Its most striking characteristic is its ability to bind reversibly oxygen and myoglobin is likely to facilitate oxygen diffusion in striated muscle fibers and also to serve as an oxygen storage within the muscle fiber.[48,49] However, its precise physiological role is still controversial. Some investigators reported that heart muscle contains multiple forms of myoglobin.[50] Whether there is a cardiac-specific myoglobin isoform in humans remains to be demonstrated. The current myoglobin assays cannot discriminate between myoglobin released from the human heart or from human skeletal muscle, and, therefore, myoglobin is not heart-specific.

MYOGLOBIN AS AN EARLY MARKER
FOR MYOCARDIAL INFARCTION

In the mid-seventies the first radioimmunoassays for measurement of myoglobin were developed[51] and became commercially available. It soon turned out that myoglobin is rapidly released after myocardial damage.[51] Since then it is an established early marker for AMI. But its determination remained only of scientific interest, because radioimmunoassays are not suitable for use in the emergency hospital laboratory. Today rapid, quantitative, and automated assays are available (immunonephelometry, immunoturbidimetry, rapid enzymimmunoassays) for "stat" determination which measure the myoglobin concentration in a sample within a few minutes.[52,53] A semiquantitative whole-blood assay also allows bedside myoglobin measurement. There are no methodological restrictions for the routine use of myoglobin any longer.

Myoglobin is markedly more sensitive than CK and CKMB activities during the first hours after the onset of chest pain (see Fig. 5.9).[53,54] It usually starts to rise within 2-4 hours after the onset of chest pain and myoglobin is detectable in all AMI patients between 6-10 hours from chest pain onset.[53,54] Its biological half-life time is only about 10-15 minutes[55] and myoglobin is rapidly cleared from the serum by the kidneys. Peak values are found in patients with early reperfusion of the infarct-related coronary artery within 7 hours from AMI onset. In all other AMI patients peaks are observed thereafter, and myoglobin returns into the reference interval usually within 24-36 hours after the onset of AMI

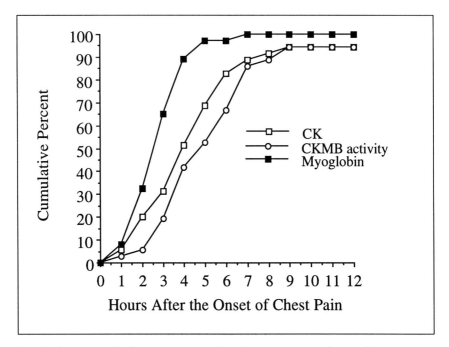

Fig. 5.9. Frequency distribution of times to first above the upper reference limit increased myoglobin, CKMB- and CK activities of 37 patients with acute myocardial infarction. The differences between myoglobin and CK or CKMB activity were significant.

(see Fig. 5.10). Myoglobin release correlates with infarct size.[56,57] Non-Q wave infarctions usually have smaller myoglobin peaks as compared to the Q wave infarctions. The rapid disappearance of myoglobin in uncomplicated AMI makes this analyte very suitable to detect a reinfarction in patients in whom chest pain reoccurs.[57]

Myoglobin is an excellent marker for ruling out an AMI in a patient admitted for chest pain.[53,54] Ideally, determinations should be carried out upon patient admission, then after 2, 4, and 6 hours. If myoglobin is still within the reference interval 8 hours after the onset of chest pain, an AMI can be ruled out with near certainty. Myoglobin was found to be a strong independent predictor of AMI in patients with symptoms of short duration, which was particularly useful in patients with an equivocal ECG at hospital admission.[58] After 12 hours, the myoglobin peak concentration may already have been passed, its efficiency drops considerably and is markedly lower than that of CKMB. CKMB determination should be preferred in patients admitted later than 10 hours from chest

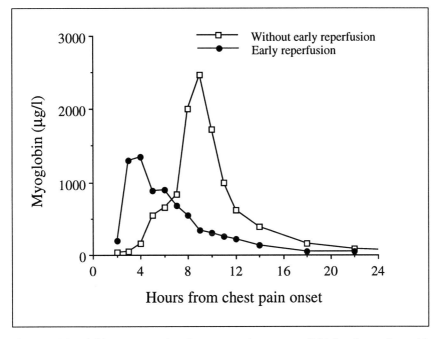

Fig. 5.10. Myoglobin concentration time courses in a myocardial infarction patient with and without early reperfusion of the infarct-related coronary artery. Both patients suffered an anterior Q-wave myocardial infarction. Both were treated with intravenous recombinant tissue-type plasminogen activator 2 hours after the onset of infarct-related symptoms.

pain onset, because myoglobin may already have normalized at the time of hospital admission.

Despite its lack of heart specificity, myoglobin is also very useful for ruling in AMI early after the onset of chest pain,[53,58] because in the nontraumatic chest pain patient admitted to the emergency department skeletal muscle damage is rare enough not to markedly influence the diagnostic efficiency of myoglobin in this patient population and missing the diagnosis AMI is the real problem for the physicians in the atypical patient. Myoglobin specificity in nontraumatic chest pain patients was reported to be in the range of that of CKMB.[53] But myoglobin should not be used for AMI testing in patients after resuscitation or with renal failure.

MONITORING OF THROMBOLYTIC THERAPY

Early reperfusion of the infarct-related coronary artery, either spontaneous or therapeutically induced by thrombolytic agents or acute PTCA, leads to a markedly more rapid and higher rate of increase and earlier peak values (see Fig. 5.10). Patients with and without early reperfusion may be reliably differentiated. Criteria based on the early rate of myoglobin increase or the relative increase over time were evaluated using acutely performed serial coronary angiographies to assess the patency of the infarct related coronary artery (see Table 5.3). In Table 5.3 only criteria are given which are based on the early rate or relative increase of myoglobin. The assessment of time to myoglobin peak values is not very useful, because the discrimination of patients with and without reperfusion is only possible at a time point when it is too late to salvage myocardium. If concomitant skeletal muscle damage can be excluded clinically, myoglobin is tendentiously the best biochemical marker to assess reperfusion noninvasively,[17] because its diagnostic performance is less susceptible to changes in the threshold value used than that of other markers.[19]

Table 5.3. Suggested myoglobin criteria for the discrimination between myocardial infarction patients with and without reperfusion

Suggested Threshold	Sensitivity	Specificity	Patency defined as
Relative increase ≥2 in 15-60 minutes after start of therapy* (ref. 59)	0.71 – 1.0	0.89 – 1.0	TIMI grade 2 or 3
Relative increase ≥3 in 30 minutes after start of therapy* (ref. 19,60)	0.81 – 0.95	0.61 – 1.0	TIMI grade 2 or 3
Slope > 150 µg/L/h (ref. 19,60)	0.82 – 0.94	0.48 – 0.88	TIMI grade 2 or 3
Relative increase ≥4 in 90 minutes after start of therapy* (ref. 19)	0.75 – 0.79	0.63 – 0.82	TIMI grade 3

* For example, a relative increase >2 means a twofold increase compared to baseline values before start of thrombolytic therapy in a given time period.
   Definition of the perfusion of the infarct-related coronary artery in the Thrombolysis in Myocardial Infarction (TIMI) trial (61):
   Grade 0 = no perfusion; grade 1 = penetration of the contrast material without perfusion; grade 2 = partial perfusion; grade 3 = complete perfusion

DIAGNOSIS OF PERIOPERATIVE MYOCARDIAL INFARCTION IN CORONARY ARTERY BYPASS GRAFTING (CABG)

Myoglobin is an early marker of perioperative myocardial infarction in patients undergoing elective CABG.[62-64] The myoglobin time course allows to differentiate patients with and without myocardial infarction several hours earlier than other markers, such as CKMB or troponins. Myoglobin concentrations in patients without perioperative myocardial infarction increase with aortic unclamping after reperfusion of the heart, peak usually after 1 hour and decrease to almost baseline values within 4 hours. By contrast, myoglobin concentrations in patients with perioperative myocardial infarction further increase after 1 hour after aortic unclamping (see Fig. 5.11). Patients with and without infarction can be discriminated as early as 3 hours after aortic unclamping.[62] Because of its short half-life in the circulation myoglobin also allows to recognize the time point of infarction onset more accurately than other markers.

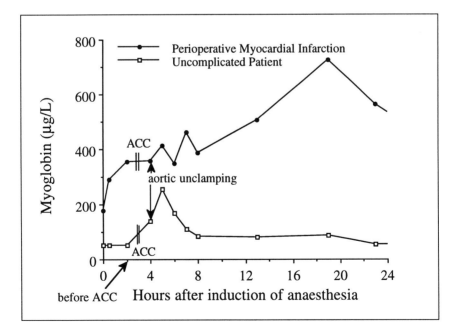

Fig. 5.11. Myoglobin concentration time courses in two representative patients undergoing elective aortocoronary bypass grafting, one with and one without perioperative myocardial infarction. Abbreviations: ACC = aortic crossclamping. Time: 0 = before anesthesia.

The concomitant skeletal muscle damage in CABG patients due to the preparation of peripheral veins, median sternotomy, or the preparation of the internal mammary artery is usually small and negligible as a source of false positive myoglobin results. Myoglobin measurements in coronary sinus blood samples[63] identified the myocardium as the major source of myoglobin release in CABG patients. However, when using alternative bypass vessels, such as the right gastroepiploic artery or the inferior epigastric artery, the surgical skeletal muscle injury is greater and myoglobin results must be assessed with caution. In these patients clearly heart-specific markers are to be preferred for diagnostic purposes.

MYOGLOBIN IN PATIENTS WITH UNSTABLE ANGINA PECTORIS

Elevated myoglobin concentrations have been reported in patients with unstable angina, perhaps reflecting small areas of myocardial muscle fiber death undetected by CKMB activity measurements.[65,66] Information on the prognostic significance of myoglobin release in these patients is limited and restricted to the development of in-hospital complications[66] which are more frequent in the patients with myoglobin increase. However, from a practical point of view it seems to be somewhat problematic to assess borderline or slight increases in myoglobin, a not heart-specific marker, in critically ill patients in whom it is not always possible to rule out skeletal muscle damage with near certainty. Therefore it is advisable to use more cardiac-specific markers for risk stratification in patients with unstable angina.

SPECIFICITY OF MYOGLOBIN

Heart and skeletal muscle are the only sources of myoglobin release. Damage to the skeletal muscles, either via trauma, surgery, or diseases, such as degenerative or inflammatory conditions, hypo- and hyperthermia, hypoxia, or alcohol abuse, also elevate myoglobin in serum.[67] Only extraordinary, unaccustomed physical exercise leads to an increase in myoglobin serum concentrations above the upper limit of the reference interval, particularly in untrained individuals. Uncomplicated intramuscular injections rarely cause false positive myoglobin results.[67] Myoglobin is also rarely elevated after cardiac catheterization. Because myoglobin is cleared from the circulation by the kidneys, patients with a decreased glomerular filtration rate from low perfusion or renal failure also can have elevated myoglobin levels.[68]

Fortunately, the problem of false positive myoglobin results is not as great as it may seem at first glance, particularly when assessing myoglobin concentrations in the nontraumatic chest pain patient (see above). The causes of such false positive results can be usually ruled out or identified easily from the clinical history, and serum urea nitrogen (BUN) and creatinine allow to assess the renal function in a patient.

OTHER APPLICATIONS

Assessment of skeletal muscle damage

Myoglobin can also be used to assess skeletal muscle injury, for example in patients with muscular dystrophies or muscle damage from electric accidents. Myoglobin increases and peaks earlier than CK. Myoglobin may also be used to assess the training status in athletes.[69,70] After a defined work load the myoglobin release from skeletal muscles is dependent on the adaptation of the muscle to the tested exercise.[70]

Assessment of the risk for the development of acute renal failure in patients with extensive skeletal muscle damage

After extensive skeletal muscle damage myoglobin concentrations are increased in urine. In patients with myocardial infarction the amount of the damaged muscle is usually too small to increase urine myoglobin.[71] In patients with rhabdomyolysis or multiple injured patients a low myoglobin clearance in the presence of high serum myoglobin concentrations indicates a high risk for the development of acute renal failure.[71] In contrast, patients with high serum myoglobin concentrations and clearances ($\geq$ 4 ml/min) have adequate renal function. Low myoglobin clearances in advance of overt renal failure indicate the need for more aggressive treatment.[71]

CARDIAC CONTRACTILE PROTEINS

Although new methods for measuring CKMB isoenzyme and its isoforms could considerably improve the diagnostic sensitivity of CKMB, there are fundamental problems with CKMB as a myocardial marker that cannot be solved by the most sophisticated methods. The CKMB content of normal myocardium is small; CKMB is not a heart-specific marker; and CKMB is detectable in the reference populations. In the final analysis CK isoenzymes and isoforms, LDH isoenzymes, and myoglobin are not sufficiently heart-specific. Therefore investigators looked for new absolutely cardiac-specific and sensitive markers. Cardiac contractile and regulatory proteins are among the most abundant proteins in cardiomyocytes, and, therefore several research groups developed immunoassays for the measurement of cardiac contractile and regulatory proteins and focused their interest on the use of myofibrillar proteins as markers for detecting myocardial damage. It was also expected that myocardial necrosis might be more accurately quantified by measurement of structurally bound muscle proteins than by measurement of cardiac enzymes.

BIOCHEMISTRY

All muscular contraction is based on a complex intracellular contractile apparatus. These proteins are highly organized in striated muscles, which leads to the typical striation pattern in histological slice images. The basic components of the contractile apparatus in striated muscles is the sarcomere. This structure is composed of a geometric arrangement of myosin-containing thick filaments surrounded by a hexagonal array of thin filaments. Thin filaments contain actin filaments and the troponin-tropomyosin regulatory complex (see Fig. 5.12). Differences in the activity patterns of slow- and fast-twitch skeletal muscle and heart muscle are reflected in the characteristics of their myofibrillar proteins; myosin, actin, tropomyosin, troponin I (TnI), troponin C (TnC), and troponin T (TnT). All exist in polymorphic forms that are characteristic of the muscle type from which the proteins are derived.

Proteins of the thin filament

Actin

Actin (MW 43 kDa) is the principal component of thin filaments. Actin filaments consist of two strands of globular molecule chains twisted in the form of a helix (see Fig. 5.12). These pseudodouble helical filaments have a pitch of approximately 13 actin monomers per turn. More than 20% of all cellular protein in striated muscle fibers is actin.

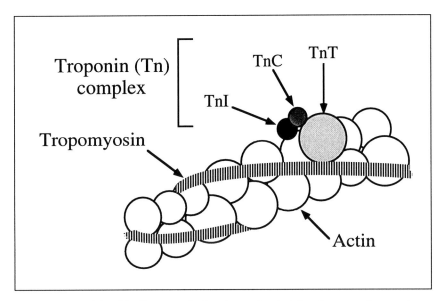

Fig. 5.12. Part of the thin filament of striated muscles showing the troponin complex.

Troponin-tropomyosin complex

In addition to actin, the thin filament also contains complexes of tropomyosin and troponin.[72] On the double-helical actin filament a troponin-tropomyosin complex is associated with each repeating region of 7 actin monomers (see Fig. 5.12; molar ratio for actin:tropomyosin:troponin of 7:1:1). Each troponin-tropomyosin complex contains four distinct polypeptides: tropomyosin and the three proteins of the troponin complex (TnI, TnT, TnC).

Tropomyosin (MW 66 kDa) is a rigid rod-shaped protein, composed of two identical α-helical chains (coiled-coil dimers of α helices). It lies in the long, pitched grooves on either side of the actin filament, and is thought to act as a "stiffener" for the filament. Tropomyosin coiled coil makes contact with seven actin monomers, as well as with neighboring tropomyosins through head-to-tail contacts. It is thought that tropomyosin sterically blocks the interaction of actin and myosin at low intracellular calcium concentrations. As the calcium concentrations are raised, the tropomyosin molecules shift their position slightly, which allows the myosin to interact with actin molecules.

Another major unit involved in calcium regulation in striated muscle is troponin complex. The troponin complex comprises three polypeptides[72] and regulates the calcium-mediated interaction of actin and myosin. The troponins are not present in smooth muscle.

1. Troponin T (TnT, MW 37 kDa) is an asymmetric protein with a globular C-terminal domain. It has a binding site for tropomyosin and is thought to be responsible for binding the troponin complex to tropomyosin.[73] The tail of TnT binds to tropomyosin and is thought to be responsible for positioning the complex on the thin filament.

2. Troponin I (TnI, MW 24 kDa) is a basic globular protein. It is the troponin complex subunit that prevents contraction in the absence of calcium and TnC by inhibiting actomyosin ATPase and thereby blocks myosin movement. This prevents the coupling of actin and myosin.

3. Troponin C (TnC, MW 18 kDa) is a dumb-bell-shaped protein with two globular domains connected by a long central helix. It binds calcium and is responsible for regulating the process of thin filament activation during skeletal and heart muscle contraction.[74] TnC can bind up to four calcium ions, and subsequently relieves the inhibition of actin-myosin interaction by inducing a steric shift and reversing the inhibitory activity of troponin I.

Proteins of the thick filament

The thick filament appears to be the major element in energy transduction and strength development. The major components of thick filaments are myosin molecules. The thick filaments are composed by about 400 aggregated molecules of myosin. About 50% of the total protein of striated muscles is myosin. Myosin molecules are highly asymmetric hexametric proteins (MW approximately 500 kDa; length 120 nm) and appear as a long α-helical section attached at the N-terminus to a globular head. Myosin molecules consist in their monomeric form of two heavy chains (MHC, MW approximately 230 kDa each) and four light chains (MLC). The MLC can be further subdivided into two alkali (essential) myosin light chains (MLC-1, molecular weight approximately 27 kDa each) and two regulatory light chains (MLC-2, molecular weight approximately 20 kDa each).

Myosin heavy chains (MHC)

The heavy chains consist of a long α-helical section attached to a globular head.[75,76] In the intact myosin molecule, the long α-helices of two heavy chains coil around each other to form the rodlike tail from which two heads project. Each of these heads is a complex of the globular head of one heavy chain with one molecule of each type of light chain. The MHC is the main component of the sarcomeric thick filament. The body of the natural thick filament is composed of some hundreds of myosin tails packed together in a regular staggered array from which the myosin heads project. Each head has an actin binding site and exhibits actin-activated ATPase activity that hydrolyzes adenosine triphosphate (ATP), thereby providing the chemical energy that is transduced into mechanical force. The velocity of shortening of a particular fiber is directly proportional to its ATPase activity which is, in turn, strongly correlated with the MHC-type composition. The isomyosins are structurally and enzymatically different. The ATPase activity of myosin is correlated with the speed of muscle shortening.

Myosin light chains (MLC)

The 4 MLC are associated with the two myosin heads. The bound light chains consist of a pair of regulatory MLC (MLC-2) and a pair of alkali (essential) MLC (MLC-1). One MLC-1 and one MLC-2 subunit are associated with the globular head region of each MHC. Although the role of the light chains is poorly understood, their location near the hinge region suggests that they may be involved in modulating interactions between myosin and actin.[75,76] Both MLC-types participate in the regulation of the interaction of actin and myosin predominantly by modulating changes in calcium flux. The two MLC-2 are phosphorylatable, allowing the myosin head to interact with an actin filament after phosphorylation, and thereby MLC-2 are involved in initiating muscle contraction.

Model of contractility

The essence of a muscle fiber is to be an engine, taking the chemical free energy of ATP and converting it into mechanical work. The sliding filament model of muscle contraction[77] postulates that the force of contraction is generated by cyclic interactions of myosin heads with the actin subunits of the thin filament (cross bridge formation). Energy for this process is derived from the hydrolysis of ATP by the actomyosin ATPase. In resting muscle, actin-myosin interactions are prevented by the troponin/tropomyosin complex. In the absence of calcium, tropomyosin would be positioned such that one step in the actomyosin-ATPase cycle is inhibited, whereas in the presence of calcium a shift in tropomyosin's position would remove the inhibition. Electrical depolarization of a striated muscle fiber leads to an increase in intracellular calcium concentration. Calcium binds to TnC, causing a conformational change of troponin-tropomyosin complex, which leads to derepression of actin-myosin interactions. Myosin heads bind to actin filaments. Subsequently the myosin heads undergo a conformational change that causes the myosin heads to "walk" along actin filaments (translation of 5-10 nm between filaments), which results in muscle fiber contraction. Muscle contraction involves sliding of constant length filaments relative to one another.

Polymorphic forms of contractile and regulatory proteins in heart and skeletal muscle

The functional differences between the muscular types are based on important structural differences. The polymorphic forms of myofibrillar proteins of striated muscle are among other factors responsible for the different contractile properties of striated muscle types. They are derived from different genes and vary in their tissue distribution, especially between cardiac and skeletal muscle. The tissue-specific isoforms differ in structure and functional properties, and consequently these antigens may be differentiated by immunologic methods. However, gene regulation of contractile proteins is complex. Striking is the degree to which cardiac, slow- and fast-twitch skeletal muscle genes are coexpressed or have "overlapping" expression, particularly between myocardium and slow-twitch skeletal muscle fibers. Yet, cardiac MLC, cardiac β-type MHC, which is the predominant MHC-type in human adult healthy and diseased myocardium, cardiac α-actin, cardiac tropomyosin, as well as cardiac TnC are coexpressed in slow-twitch skeletal muscle fibers.[74,78-82] Therefore, these proteins cannot provide absolute cardiac-specificity despite the application of highly specific monoclonal antibodies in assays. There remain only two candidates for heart-specific markers, cTnI and cTnT. Troponin I and troponin T exist in three different isoforms with a unique structure, one for slow-twitch skeletal muscle, one for fast-twitch skeletal muscle, and one for cardiac muscle.[83,84] The three isoforms are encoded by three different genes. cTnI has an extra 31 amino acid residues at the N-terminus and its amino acid sequence shows about 40% dissimilarity from both other isoforms.[84] cTnT differs only by 6-11 amino acid residues from its skeletal muscle isoforms. In comparison of the cTnT amino acid sequence with the sequences of both skeletal TnT isoforms, only 10-30% of its amino acid sequence show low homology with skeletal TnT isoforms.[83] Therefore it is more difficult to produce cardiac-specific anti cTnT antibodies.

ACTIN

Actin (MW 43 kDa) is encoded by a multigene family in mammals. Actins from fast and slow-twitch skeletal muscle are identical. Therefore only two different sarcomeric actins have been identified, the α-skeletal and the α-cardiac isoforms, which are encoded by two different genes. Both are distinguishable from nonmuscular and myoblast precursor actins (β- and γ-actins). Differences between the primary sequences of α-skeletal and α-cardiac actin isoforms have been reported. Despite the high degree of homology between these actins, important differences exist within the essential peptide sequence that constitutes the myosin binding domain. However, analytically these isoforms behave very similar (difference of four amino acids at the amino terminus), and it is very difficult to distinguish between them at the protein level.[85] Furthermore, the α-cardiac actin gene is expressed in both heart and skeletal muscle, and α-skeletal actin is the major isoform of all of normal, hypertrophied and failing human hearts (review in ref. 81). As such α-cardiac actin is not a suitable candidate for the development of an assay specific for myocardial damage.

Clinical results

The data on actin in serum of patients with acute coronary syndromes are very limited. Circulating α-cardiac actin has been described in patients with AMI and unstable angina pectoris using western-blot analysis.[86] A biphasic time course was described with an increase within a few hours from chest pain onset, a first peak on the first day and a second peak 2-3 days after the attack. Alpha cardiac actin remained detectable for up to 7 days. Alpha cardiac actin was also detected in some patients with skeletal muscle damage, demonstrating the limited diagnostic specificity of this marker.

TROPOMYOSIN

The α-skeletal form of tropomyosin is identical to the cardiac form in mammals including men.[82] Thus the development of a tropomyosin assay without crossreactivity with tropomyosins isolated from skeletal muscle is not possible and it is not a good candidate for AMI-specific diagnosis.

Clinical results

Little data on tropomyosin release after AMI exist so far.[87] The initial pattern of release of tropomyosin is very similar to that of CK, being detectable within 7-8 hours after infarction. Tropomyosin reaches peak values a few hours later than CKMB and CK. In contrast to CK and CKMB, tropomyosin concentrations are still raised above normal after 72 hours and do not return to normal until 8-12 days after infarction depending on the severity of the infarct. It proved possible to measure significant increases in tropomyosin concentrations even in patients where only small increases in CK activities were present.

CARDIAC TROPONIN C

No data on a cardiac TnC assay or the TnC release after cardiac damage have been published yet. However, cardiac TnC is not a suitable candidate for the development of an assay specific for myocardial damage, because ventricular and slow-twitch skeletal TnC are identical in humans.[74]

CARDIAC TROPONIN T

Troponin T (TnT) exists in at least three isotypes, two skeletal and one cardiac (MW approximately 37 kDa) with high sequence homology. But these differences in the amino acid sequence determine the important myofilamental structural and functional properties unique to the cardiac isotype. Separate genes encode troponin from cardiac muscle, and slow-twitch and fast-twitch skeletal muscle fibers. Both cardiac and skeletal TnT are coexpressed in the fetal heart,[88] but the skeletal isotype is subsequently suppressed during the prenatal period. Controversial reports exist on the topic whether cardiac TnT (cTnT) exists in the human heart as one or two major isoforms.[88,89] In the adult human heart Anderson et al[88] have described multiple isoforms of cTnT, while Katus et al[89] found only one in normal and failing human heart. According to Anderson et al[88] skeletal muscle TnT can be reexpressed in human myocardium under conditions of cardiac stress, and human myocardium seems to have the potential to express more than one isoform of cTnT, and maturational development as well as cardiac disease alter TnT expression. These isoforms are thought to be generated by alternate splicing of a primary transcript from the same gene. Anderson et al[88] reported on at least two major isoforms of cTnT, labeled $cTnT_1$ and $cTnT_2$. These isoforms were not found in adult skeletal muscle. They have different sensitivities with regard to calcium and ATPase activity. $cTnT_1$ is the predominant form found in normal adult cardiac tissue. In patients with left ventricular failure there is an increased expression of $cTnT_2$ isoform. This is associated with a reduction of myofibrillar ATPase. Whether this contributes or is an adaptation to heart failure is not known so far.

In the human heart muscle approximately 6% (approximately 0.025 mg/g wet weight) of the total myocardial cTnT is found as a soluble, cytoplasmatic pool, which probably serves as a precursor pool for the synthesis of the troponin-complex.[90] In our own experiments we found a cytoplasmatic cTnT pool of approximately 5% (unpublished data).

cTnT is absent in the adult human skeletal muscle.[88] In fetal muscle, however, small amounts of cTnT were reported particularly in slow-twitch muscle tissue.[88] cTnT is downregulated during the prenatal period. Fortunately, this is not of clinical relevance, because there is usually no interest in measuring cTnT in fetal blood to assess myocardial injury in fetus. However, the fact that cTnT is found in small amounts in the fetal skeletal muscle may be of clinical relevance, because it has been shown that the chronically stressed skeletal muscle may revert to the expression of fetal proteins.[91] By immunofluorescence staining cTnT was found in regenerating rat adult skeletal muscle after a "cold injury" or after denervation.[92] Since the troponin complex is highly conserved throughout phylogeny, cTnT could be theoretically reexpressed also in regenerating human skeletal muscle. Whether this really occurs in humans is not sufficiently investigated so far. Recently, Bodor et al found, using immunfluorescence staining, evidence for cTnT being present in biopsies obtained from patients with polymyositis and Duchenne muscular dystrophy.[93] However, a definitive proof requires the demonstration of reexpression of cTnT on the protein level (western-blot) and mRNA level (northern-blot), which is still lacking.

The new improved, already commercially available cTnT assay shows no crossreactivity with skeletal troponins.[94] The biggest advantages of this TnT assay over CKMB and LDH assays are its cardiac-specificity (no crossreactivity with skeletal muscle TnT) and its high sensitivity for even small amounts of myocardial necrosis. Baseline levels are normally very low (concentrations in healthy individuals are below or in the range of the analytical detection limit of the assay) and elevations are substantial when myocardial damage occurs. A lot of information on the use of cTnT to diagnose acute coronary syndromes is already available.

Acute myocardial infarction (AMI)

Troponin T time course in blood after AMI
cTnT allows early and late diagnosis of AMI (long diagnostic window). Figure 5.13 shows cTnT changes compared with conventional markers and cTnI in a representative AMI patient. Concentrations of serum cTnT start increasing within a few hours after the onset of symptoms (median: 3, range: 1-10 hours).[12,95] A plateau is often observed from the second to the 5th day. The sensitivity of cTnT for detecting myocardial infarction is 100% from 10 hours to at least 5 days after the onset of chest pain. cTnT concentrations identify all Q and non-Q wave myocardial infarction during this time interval.[95,96] In contrast to the transient usefulness of CKMB measurements, the efficiency of cTnT remains 98% until 6 days after admission.[96] In many AMI patients increased cTnT concentrations beyond the 7th day allow the diagnosis based on this biochemical marker even during the second week after onset of AMI. Concentrations are increased for up to 3 weeks in some patients with late and/or high peak values. Consequently, cTnT determinations are particularly useful for a late diagnosis of myocardial infarction in AMI patients who do not seek

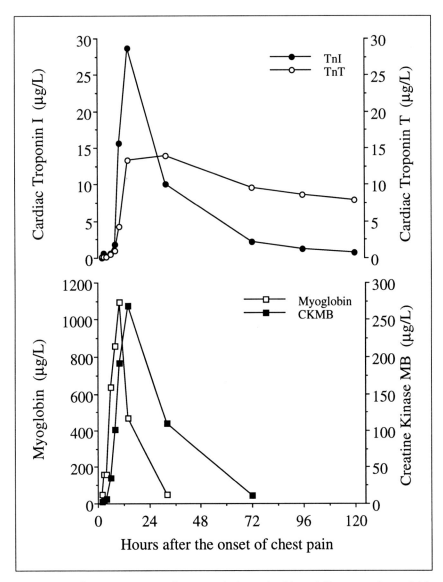

Fig. 5.13. Cardiac troponin T, cardiac troponin I, creatine kinase MB mass, and myoglobin concentration time courses in a representative patient with acute myocardial infarction without early reperfusion of the infarct-related coronary artery. This patient without early reperfusion suffered an inferior wall AMI and was treated with urokinase. Coronary angiography 12 days after AMI revealed a left ventricular ejection fraction of 47% and a 99% stenosis of the infarct-related coronary artery (Thrombolysis in Myocardial Infarction [TIMI] Trial grade 1 [penetration without] perfusion).

medical attention within the 2-3 day window during which CK and CKMB are elevated. Another striking feature of cTnT following AMI is its high relative increase compared to cTnT concentrations measured in healthy controls. A comparable increase in AMI patients has been only described for cTnI concentrations so far.[12] cTnT shows an average 100-fold increase above the upper limit of the reference interval. In patients with small AMI the time course of cTnT contrasts more strongly with the normal range than CK and LDH isoenzyme activities.[95,97] Thus, cTnT measurements are particularly useful in patients with small AMI or borderline CKMB activity in whom the diagnosis of AMI cannot be made or excluded with near certainty.

In AMI, a biphasic pattern of cTnT release with peaks at about 14 hours and 3-5 days has been demonstrated (see Fig. 5.14). These serum concentration changes of cTnT after myocardial damage are most probably explained by the intracellular compartmentalization of this protein. cTnT release reveals characteristics of both free cytosolic molecules on the first 2 days and of structurally bound constituents thereafter. The rapid loss of the cytosolic cTnT pool of damaged myocytes leads to an increase in cTnT serum concentrations within a few hours after the onset of myocardial damage. It is likely that apart from the presence of such a relatively small cytosolic pool of cardiac troponins not incorporated into the myofibrils which may serve as a source for early troponin release, also other factors contribute to the early release and early troponin peaks after myocardial infarction. A rapid degradation of troponins after a 60 minute lasting complete global myocardial ischemia with anoxia was observed in rat hearts.[98] Among myofibrillar proteins TnT and TnI appear to be particularly susceptible to calpain digestion which is a soluble calcium-dependent proteolytic system,[99] and this may contribute to the early increase in cTnT and cTnI and also to the early peaks of both proteins after myocardial damage. cTnT remains elevated for several days and shows peaks also about day 4 after the onset of AMI. This reflects continuous release of protein from disintegrating myofilaments because the half-life time of cTnT in blood is only about 2-4 hours.[90] The presence of a cytoplasmatic cTnT pool raises doubts whether short and slight cTnT increases are specific for myocyte death. That continuing release for days caused by dissociation of the contractile apparatus indicates cell death is less controversial.

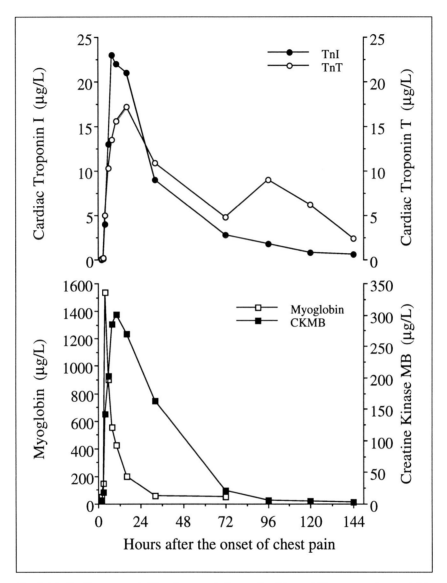

Fig. 5.14. Cardiac troponin T and troponin I, creatine kinase MB mass, and myoglobin concentration time courses in a representative patient with acute myocardial infarction and early reperfusion of the infarct-related coronary artery. This patient with early reperfusion suffered an inferior wall AMI and was treated with streptokinase. Coronary angiography 7 days after AMI revealed a left ventricular ejection fraction of 50% (good function) and an open infarct-related coronary artery (stenosis 50%, Thrombolysis in Myocardial Infarction [TIMI] Trial grade 3 [complete] perfusion).[61]

Early myocardial infarct detection

cTnT is an early marker of myocardial injury as well (see Fig. 5.15). The sensitivities of cTnT, cTnI, CK isoforms, CKMB mass, and myoglobin are roughly comparable during a 0-6-hour period after the onset of chest pain.[12] The differences in sensitivities are small and the clinical significance of differences is low. However, the sensitivities of myoglobin and CKMB mass concentrations tended to be somewhat higher during the 2-5 hour time interval. However, none of the tested parameters[12] reliably diagnose AMI within the first 3-4 hours after the onset of chest pain. Fifty percent of all AMI patients investigated had increased cTnT concentrations at 3 hours[12,96] after the onset of chest pain. cTnT is 100% sensitive from 10 hours after the onset of infarct-related symptoms until the 5th to 6th day after AMI.[95,96] Thus, cTnT is also an early marker of myocardial damage. On the other hand, cTnT concentrations measured after a 12-hour observation period in patients without recurrent chest pain could provide a simple,

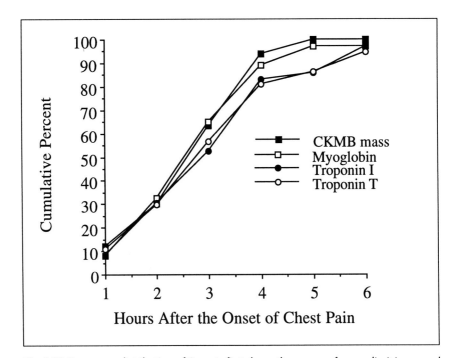

Fig. 5.15. Frequency distribution of times to first above the upper reference limit increased cardiac troponin T and troponin I, myoglobin, and CKMB mass concentrations of 37 patients with acute myocardial infarction. There were no statistical significant differences between markers.[12]

sensitive and specific diagnostic aid to exclude acute coronary syndromes and identify candidates for the early "step down" transfer from the coronary care unit—thus, resulting in more efficient and economic use of the critical care facility. A reliable, semiquantitative whole blood test for the bedside measurement of cTnT has already been developed and is available for routine use.[100]

Effects of infarct-related artery reperfusion on the release kinetics of troponin T in acute myocardial infarction patients

Reperfusion influences the release of cTnT in AMI patients.[17,19,90,95,101] In AMI patients with early reperfusion, cTnT appears in serum significantly earlier and peak values are observed significantly earlier as well. In patients who undergo thrombolytic treatment cTnT concentration changes on the first day vary highly (see Figs. 5.13 and 5.14). The appearance of cTnT in serum on day 1 after the onset of AMI depends strongly on reperfusion and on the duration of ischemia until reperfusion occurs.[90] AMI reperfusion obviously leads to a "washout" of the free cytosolic cTnT pool, resulting in a rapid increase in cTnT. By contrast, the kinetics of cTnT release after the first 38 hours after AMI is unaffected by reperfusion.

Early reperfusion

In successfully early reperfused patients, cTnT peaks within 24 hours after admission. A marked distinct peak in cTnT concentrations with a subsequent rapid decrease is found at a median time of 14 hours after the onset of chest pain in all patients with reperfused AMI within 3.5 hours after the onset of pain.[90] A second much smaller peak is observed at about the 4th day after admission to the hospital (see Fig. 5.14). cTnT appears and disappears in serum significantly earlier in patients with early reperfused AMI.

Late reperfusion or permanent occlusion

In patients without thrombolytic therapy and no spontaneous early reperfusion or failed reperfusion therapy there is no distinct cTnT peak on day 1 (see Fig. 5.13). In these patients, maximal cTnT concentrations occur several days after admission, on or about the 4th day after the onset of symptoms. The early peak is absent in patients with AMI reperfusion occurring more than 5.5 hours after the onset of pain.[90]

The effects of reperfusion on the cTnT release kinetics in AMI can be used to noninvasively assess the effectiveness of thrombolytic therapy. All patients with AMI reperfusion less than 5.5 hours after the onset of pain had ratios of peak cTnT concentration day 1 to cTnT concentration at day 4 of more than 1.0 due to a marked cTnT "washout phenomenon", whereas in patients with nonreperfused AMI this ratio is ≤1.0.[90] Similarly, in reperfused patients the ratio of cTnT 14 hours to that 38 hours after the onset of acute myocardial infarction is >1.1.[102] However, such criteria allow only a retrospective documentation of reperfusion and their clinical usefulness is very limited. Therefore, in Table 5.4 only criteria are listed for the discrimination of patients with and without reperfusion which are based on the early rate of cTnT or relative cTnT increase. These criteria were established using serial acute coronary angiographies to assess the reperfusion status of the infarct-related coronary artery.

Noninvasive estimation of infarct size

It could be demonstrated that the cTnT release in patients with AMI is related to other independent measures (left ventricular ejection fraction, scintigraphic estimates of myocardial scar) of infarct size.[103,104] The cTnT value on the 3-4 day after AMI can be used as a gross estimate of myocardial infarct size.[104] However, it remains to be shown whether in AMI patients cumulative cTnT release provides a more useful tool for noninvasive estimation of infarct size than commonly used cumulative CKMB or LDH-1 release.

Diagnosis of perioperative myocardial infarction

Diagnosis of perioperative myocardial infarction in noncardiac surgery

The most important advantage of cTnT is its cardiac-specificity, because the new assay shows no crossreactivity with skeletal TnT.[94] Thus, measurements are especially helpful in the assessment of patients with myocardial ischemia and skeletal muscle injury, e.g., after surgery. Therefore, troponins should replace CKMB measurements in the laboratory diagnosis of perioperative myocardial infarction, because cTnT and cTnI are the most useful markers to assess the presence or absence of cardiac injury in patients with skeletal muscle damage.[96,105]

Table 5.4. Suggested cardiac troponin T criteria for the discrimination
between myocardial infarction patients with and without reperfusion

Suggested Threshold	Sensitivity	Specificity	Patency defined as
Slope > 0.2 µg/L/h (ref. 17,19)	0.64 – 0.80	0.53 – 0.65	TIMI grade 2 or 3
Relative increase ≥ 6.8 in 90 minutes after start of therapy* (ref. 19)	0.70 – 0.89	0.66 – 0.83	TIMI grade 3
Slope > 0.5 µg/L/h (ref. 99)	0.83 – 0.92	1.0	TIMI grade 2 or 3

* For example, a relative increase >6.8 means a >6.8 increase compared to baseline values before start of thrombolytic therapy in a given time period.
    Definition of the perfusion of the infarct-related coronary artery in the Thrombolysis in Myocardial Infarction (TIMI) trial (61):
    Grade 0 = no perfusion; grade 1 = penetration of the contrast material without perfusion; grade 2 = partial perfusion; grade 3 = complete perfusion

Diagnosis of perioperative AMI in coronary artery bypass grafting (CABG) surgery

As for other cardiac enzymes and proteins after CABG, general reference limits of cTnT are not valid as there is inevitable cardiac tissue damage (e.g., by right atriotomy for cannulation, cardioplegic cardiac arrest, or intermittent aortic cross-clamping) occurring during the surgical procedure.[106-108] Figure 5.16 shows the cTnT time courses after CABG in a patient with PMI and in an uncomplicated patient. In PMI, cTnT concentrations start increasing with aortic unclamping, peak on or about the 4th postoperative day and remain increased until at least the 7th day after CABG surgery. In patients with PMI cTnT concentrations exceed 2.5 µg/l.[109] cTnT in patients without complications also significantly increases after reperfusion over values seen before bypass and stays increased for several days. cTnT concentrations in completely uneventful patients do not exceed 1.0 µg/L and show a biphasic release with a first peak between 4-8 hours after aortic unclamping and a second peak about 4 days after surgery.[110] The second peak is frequently less pronounced; instead, time courses often show a plateau from the first to the 4th postoperative day (see Fig. 5.16). This probably reflects myocardial cell damage from cannulation of the great vessels, which includes atrial incisions, or effect of ischemia during cardioplegia. In these patients, cTnT concentrations (peak values, duration of increase) are associated with the duration of cardiac arrest and aortic cross clamping.[107] After CABG surgery there is a third group of patients with minor perioperative myocardial damage.[107,108] cTnT in these patients is >1.0 µg/L and significantly higher than in completely uneventful patients. However, these patients do not meet the standard criteria of PMI. Nonspecific ECG changes are frequent in those patients. Perioperative myocardial cell damage seems to be much more common than has been previously recognized by changes of ECG and serum enzyme activities. In summary, cTnT reliably identifies perioperative infarction during CABG and is superior to CKMB activity, especially in diagnosing minor perioperative myocardial damage. cTnT may be very useful in assessing the effectiveness of various cardioprotective measures.

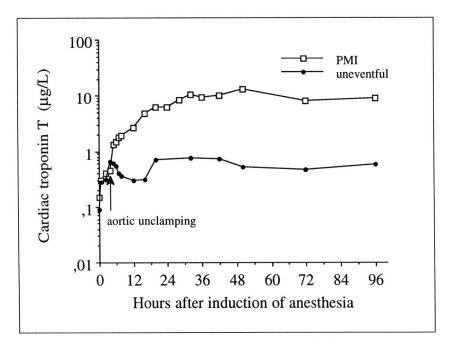

Fig. 5.16. Cardiac troponin T time courses in two patients with elective coronary artery bypass grafting, one uneventful patient and one patient with perioperative myocardial infarction.

Separate postsurgical cTnT reference intervals have to be evaluated for other cardiac surgical procedures, especially if they include cardiotomy, e.g., mitral valve surgery and CABG during the same operation. For all other cardiac surgical procedures (e.g., valve replacements in patients without coronary artery disease, corrections of malformations of the heart) PMI is fortunately a rare complication. Because of cardiotomy with surgical trauma to the heart also cTnT is not useful for PMI diagnosis in these patients.

Diagnosis of minor myocardial damage ("microinfarction") in patients with unstable angina pectoris

Increased cTnT concentrations have been described in a subgroup of patients with angina pectoris at rest (approximately 30% of patients with unstable angina Braunwald severity class III).[20,96,111] It is assumed that these patients sustained "minor myocardial damage" (or "microinfarction") which does not meet the standard AMI criteria.[20,96,111] cTnT was not detected in patients with stable angina, accelerated or subacute angina at rest. cTnT concentrations in patients with angina at rest correlated with ECG signs of myocardial ischemia. The incidence of in-hospital development of AMI and death and the long-term cardiac event rate during the subsequent months were significantly different between the groups positive and negative for cTnT. However, Katus et al[96] emphasize that the cTnT test cannot be used to screen (negative predictive value: 0.26) for the presence of severe coronary artery disease (>75% obstruction of a major coronary artery). In patients with unstable angina normal cTnT test results in serially drawn blood samples rule out AMI and "microinfarction" but do not preclude the presence of severe coronary artery disease and a poor long-term prognosis for the patient. A protein marker can only indicate acute myocardial ischemia and, thus, only indirectly indicates the state of a coronary vessel (acutely unstable coronary lesions). On the other hand, increased cTnT concentrations in patients with unstable angina indicate recently developed severe coronary artery narrowing with high specificity (0.85).[96] In patients with unstable angina, cTnT measurements are a useful indicator of cardiac risk during hospitalization and the subsequent months.[20,111] By serial sampling in patients with unstable angina Ravkilde et al found that the prognostic value of CKMB mass, myosin light chains, and cTnT is equivalent.[20] All tested markers were independent risk factors for the development of cardiac events. However, in this study marker protein increase could not add additional prognostic information to ECG, that are ECG signs for myocardial ischemia at rest.[20] However, recent data on risk stratification in patients with acute coronary syndromes of the GUSTO-IIa and FRISC trials[112,113] demonstrated that cTnT is an independent risk factor (higher values are associated with increasing rates of cardiac events) and that cTnT concentrations were significantly more strongly associated with mortality than CKMB mass concentrations. The admission cTnT concentration provided the most important risk stratification. Currently there is no doubt that patients with chest pain who tested positive for cTnT at hospital admission have a much worse prognosis than patients who tested negative. Current studies evaluate the cost-effectiveness of cTnT testing for patients' outcome, time to treatment, and length of stay in the hospital.

cTnT concentrations after invasive-cardiological procedures

Percutaneous transluminal coronary angioplasty (PTCA) and related procedures

PTCA

PTCA is a method used frequently to dilate stenotic coronary arteries. After PTCA, cTnT is a sensitive marker for determining whether myocardial injury is present or not.[114,115] In uncomplicated PTCA patients, cTnT does not increase in serum over a baseline measure (see Fig. 5.17). However, angiographically visible occlusion of smaller side-branches next to the site of the dilated stenosis, although symptomless, may lead to a slight increase in cTnT. In these patients and other patients with minor complications (prolonged chest pain, ECG documented episodes of myocardial ischemia) which do not fulfill standard WHO AMI criteria cTnT concentrations after PTCA usually stay <1.5 µg/l depending on baseline values within the reference interval. Reocclusion of a successfully dilated stenosis causes a marked rise in cTnT similar to other AMI patients (see Fig. 5.17). Prolonged release of cTnT into blood reflects more severe damage to myocytes than simple leakage of CKMB. The extent of myocardial damage after PTCA

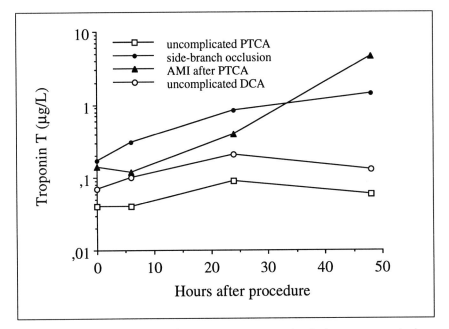

Fig. 5.17. Cardiac troponin T after percutaneous transluminal coronary angioplasty (PTCA) or directional coronary atherectomy (DCA). Abbreviation: Acute Myocardial Infarction (AMI)

can be graded by cTnT measurements,[114] which could be a valuable diagnostic aid to the decision process when to discharge a patient from the hospital after PTCA.

Coronary rotational ablation, directional coronary atherectomy

According to first results the percentage of patients with increased cTnT following these interventions is not markedly higher than after PTCA.

Defibrillation threshold tests during implantation of intracardiac defibrillators

Increases in cTnT were found after this intervention. cTnT release correlated with the duration of fibrillation.

Radiofrequency catheter ablation therapy of cardiac rhythm disturbances

Radiofrequency energy produces cell damage by resistive tissue heating. The purpose, for example, is to destroy accessory pathways which are responsible for episodes of tachycardia. After such interventions all myocardial proteins including cTnT frequently increase in blood. There is a relation between increase in markers and the radiofrequency cumulated power and application time.

Nonischemic myocardial damage

Myocarditis

The high sensitivity and cardiospecificity of the cTnT assay suggest that cTnT measurements might discern myocardial muscle damage in myocarditis patients. In murine autoimmune myocarditis Bachmaier et al[116] found that cTnT is a more sensitive marker for the disease than CKMB. Elevations clearly indicated myocarditis, but negative results do not exclude the presence of the disease. In animals or patients with mainly interstitial inflammatory infiltrates myocyte necrosis is not prominent and marker elevations may be absent. Increased cTnT concentrations in patients with confirmed myocarditis have been described.[96,117] Increases in cTnT could be documented in patients with biopsy verified myocarditis in whom CK and CKMB were within the reference interval. The current data suggest that cTnT is a more sensitive parameter than CK and CKMB for detection of myocardial damage in acute myocarditis.

Slightly increased concentrations of cTnT can also be found in a subgroup of patients with dilated cardiomyopathy, which is related to a worse prognosis compared with patients without detectable cTnT. This is probably explained by the ongoing loss of cardiomyocytes.

Rejection of the transplanted heart

Walpoth et al demonstrated in a rat model of heart transplantation that cTnT release during episodes of cardiac rejection was correlated to the severity of rejection assessed by histological examination.[118] This correlation was closer than those for CK and CKMB activities. After orthotopic heart transplantation in men cTnT moderately increases. Peak values (approximately 2-5 µg/L) are observed about 1 week after transplantation. In contrast to CKMB, cTnT remains detectable in these patients for at least 6 weeks even without episodes of rejection.[119] The reasons for this are not known so far. However, this behavior of cTnT makes the marker less useful for the detection of episodes of rejection than markers which more rapidly normalize after surgery, because frequent blood sampling is necessary to recognize a new increase in cTnT. A principal limitation of all intramyocardial proteins when used for the early detection of rejection episodes is that they only increase when myocardial damage has already occurred.

However, circulating cTnT can also be used to assess the heart in a potential heart transplant donor.[120] Brain death may induce myocardial dysfunction, and the quality of the donor's heart is considered an important prognostic factor in heart transplantation. In contrast to CKMB, an elevated cTnT was associated with a severe decrease in left ventricular function, and donor cTnT predicts subsequent inotropic requirements in the immediate postoperative period following transplantation. Donor cTnT may be a useful predictor of early allograft dysfunction and may influence the decision to use the heart for transplantation.

Heart contusion

cTnT measurements are particularly useful in the assessment of cardiac injury in the presence of skeletal muscle damage (see above). Serial cTnT measurements are a valuable aid in the diagnosis of heart contusion.[121] cTnT measurements are particularly useful to determine heart contusion in the patient with isolated chest trauma. However, it remains to be demonstrated if patients with increase in cTnT have a worse prognosis than patients without. In the multiply injured patient the diagnosis of heart contusion, apart from the obvious, clinically diagnosed cases, may be of little prognostic relevance. Nonetheless, if the clinician orders a marker to assess myocardial injury, cTnT and cTnI should replace less cardiac-specific CKMB measurements as a criterion in the laboratory diagnosis of blunt heart trauma.

Diagnostic specificity of cardiac troponin T

The latest and currently commercially available version of the cTnT assay shows no crossreactivity with skeletal troponins. Currently there are no known analytical interferences causing false positive results,[94] and this assay is analytically specific for cTnT. The only considerable analytical interference may result from the administration of high doses of biotin (e.g., in the patient with hemodialysis), which may cause false negative results; blood samples should be drawn at least 8 hours after the last biotin dose.

The diagnostic specificity of cTnT for myocardial injury is not fully delineated so far. Recently, serum cTnT concentrations of patients with polymyositis and dermatomyositis have been reported by Kobayashi et al.[122] The purpose of this study was to demonstrate cardiac involvement (myocarditis) in these patients. cTnT could not be detected in the serum of patients with rheumatoid arthritis or systemic lupus erythematosus. By contrast, 27% of patients with polymyositis or dermatomyositis had serum cTnT above normal. However, the majority of these patients showed no other signs of cardiac involvement. These results and similar studies on troponins in myopathy[123] are frequently cited when questioning the specificity of cTnT as a marker for cardiac injury. However, it must be stressed that in all studies on this topic published so far the investigators used a cTnT assay which showed some residual crossreactivity with skeletal TnT and the clinical relevance of these reports has to be questioned. We could not detect cTnT by western-blotting in skeletal muscle despite clear histological alterations in a murine model of Duchenne muscular dystrophy so far (preliminary own unpublished results). Similarly, we could not detect cTnT by western-blotting in skeletal muscle biopsies of patients with mitochondrial myopathies so far (preliminary own unpublished results). But clearly this issue also has to be investigated in skeletal muscle biopsies obtained from patients with Duchenne or Becker muscular dystrophy, polymositis, or dermatomyositis. Therefore, as long as the topic of whether cTnT may be reexpressed in skeletal muscle of patients with myopathies involving unremitting degeneration and regeneration has not been fully delineated, serum cTnT concentrations in patients with myopathies must be assessed with caution.

Increased cTnT with cTnI within the reference interval has been reported in patients with chronic maintenance hemodialysis who showed no clinical, ECG, echocardiographic, or other signs of acute myocardial injury.[124,125] Whether cTnT positive patients more frequently showed renal myopathy than cTnT negative patients was not reported in these investigations. Again in these studies a cTnT assay with residual crossreactivity with skeletal troponin T was used and these results might not reflect the true situation. However, also when measuring cTnT with the new generation cTnT assay increased cTnT and cTnI are found in about 3-5% of patients undergoing chronic maintenance hemodialysis. This obviously reflects the high prevalence of coronary artery disease and myocardial ischemia in these patients. However, there are an additional approximately 20% of patients who have elevated cTnT with normal cTnI. Currently Katus and coworkers investigate whether these patients are a high risk subgroup for the development of cardiac events. Thus far, he and his coworkers could not demonstrate cTnT by western-blotting in skeletal muscle specimens obtained during renal transplantation (personal communication).

Clinical use of cardiac troponin T—Summary

The following proposed indications for usage of cardiac TnT measurements are derived from current clinical results with the new cTnT assay:

1. *Acute myocardial infarction:* During the early stages of myocardial infarction cTnT measurements are particularly useful to assess the extent of myocardial damage in: (1) patients with concomitant skeletal muscle injury—for example, after cardiopulmonary resuscitation, direct-current countershock therapy, or in patients presenting with chest pain after heavy physical exercise and (2) patients with borderline CKMB. A single cTnT measurement on the 3rd to 5th day allows to grossly assess the amount of damaged myocardium.

2. *Late diagnosis of myocardial infarction:* cTnT measurements are useful in myocardial infarction patients who do not seek medical attention within the 48-72 hour period during which CK and CKMB are elevated. The diagnostic efficiency of cTnT remains 98% until 6 days after the onset of infarct-related symptoms.

3. *Monitoring the effectiveness of thrombolytic therapy in AMI patients:* The collection of two blood samples (before, and 60-90 minutes after start of thrombolytic therapy) for the calculation of slope or relative cTnT increase is recommended (see above).

4. *Risk stratification in patients with acute coronary syndromes.*

5. *Assessment of myocardial injury after PTCA and related procedures.*

6. *Diagnosis of perioperative AMI including CABG—surgery.*

7. *Diagnosis of blunt heart trauma.*

8. *Diagnosis of myocarditis.*

For reasons outlined above, currently serum cTnT has to be interpreted with caution in patients with chronic myopathies, renal diseases, and multiple organ failure.

CARDIAC TROPONIN I

Cardiac troponin I (cTnI) is uniquely located in the myocardium where it is the only TnI isotype form present. It is distributed uniformly throughout atrial and ventricular chambers.[126] Also on the basis of evidence obtained by molecular cloning, in human heart muscle only a single TnI isoform exists which contains a specific N-terminal 31 amino acid sequence that is lacking in skeletal muscle TnI isoforms.[127] cTnI remains the only TnI isoform expressed in human myocardium even during chronic disease processes.[126,127] Throughout ontogeny cTnI is not expressed in skeletal muscle.[128] Fetal myocardium of humans contains slow-twitch TnI (predominant in fetal heart) and cTnI initially, but after the ninth postnatal month only cTnI is expressed in the human heart.[127-129] cTnI has not been detected in other tissues apart from the heart at any developmental stage or in diseased skeletal muscle.[128-130] Thus, the presence of cTnI in the circulation above the reference limit is highly specific for myocardial injury.

Experimental results indicate the presence of a cytoplasmic precursor pool of unassembled TnI.[131] Recently the cytoplasmatic fraction was quantified, and it was found that it amounted to approximately 3-5% of the total cTnI content (which is approximately 4 mg/g wet weight) in human myocardium.[105,132] Therefore it is, similar to cTnT, questionable whether slight cTnI increases of short duration really reflect myocardial cell death (see troponin T). There is a approximately 13-fold greater concentration of cTnI than CKMB in the heart.[132]

Detection of acute myocardial infarction, monitoring of thrombolytic therapy, and estimation of infarct size by measurement of cTnI

Detection of cTnI in serum after AMI has first been described by Cummins and coworkers[126] by use of a radioimmunoassay. Most authors observed first increases above normal levels between 3 and 8 hours (see Fig. 5.15) after onset of AMI specific symptoms in humans[105,126,132] and experimental animals in parallel to CKMB[133]

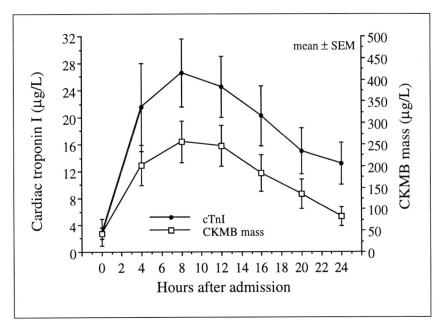

Fig. 5.18. Cardiac troponin I and CKMB mass concentration time courses in AMI patients. Data given as mean ± SEM (n = 18).

(see Fig. 5.18). We also found no difference between the early sensitivities of cTnT, and cTnI, and myoglobin and CKMB mass tended to be somewhat more sensitive only during the 2-5 hour period after chest pain onset (see Fig. 5.15).[12] Peak serum values are reached after 12-24 hours (depending on reperfusion), with cTnI concentrations returning to normal after 120-450 hours depending on AMI size. cTnI release in AMI patients is related to scintigraphic estimates of myocardial scar.[134] As with myosin light chain-1 and cTnT a biphasic release profile can be observed in many patients, that may be caused by two different pools of cTnI, i.e., a cytoplasmatic and a structurally bound compartment.[126] Similar to cTnT, also other factors apart from the presence of a relatively small cytoplasmatic pool must be responsible for the early cTnI peak values which occur in parallel to CKMB peaks (for possible mechanisms involved see troponin T).

The release profile of cTnI from the infarcted myocardium is influenced by successful coronary artery recanalization.[105,135,136] In successfully reperfused patients with Q-wave or non-Q-wave infarction the peak values are reached earlier. In Q-wave AMI with early reperfusion the cTnI peaks are usually higher, and the return to normal concentrations is accelerated when compared to nonsuccessfully treated or untreated patients (see Figs. 5.13, 5.14, 5.19, 5.20). cTnI criteria (slope, relative increase) for the early discrimination between patients with and without reperfusion of the infarct-related coronary artery are currently established with acute coronary angiography controlled studies, but the results are not yet available.

Comparison of cTnI and cTnT time courses after AMI

cTnI increases and mostly peaks in parallel to cTnT (see Figs. 5.13-5.15).[12,105] cTnI and cTnT usually peak in parallel except for patients without reperfusion in whom cTnI peaks about one day and cTnT approximately 3-4 days after onset of AMI.[105,136] Troponin peak values correlate closely.[105] In contrast to cTnI, cTnT mostly shows a second, usually smaller, peak about day 4 after AMI. Both stay increased for at least 4-5 days. cTnT tends to stay increased longer than cTnI. cTnT sensitivity on the 7th day after AMI was significantly higher than that of cTnI.[105] In general, cTnT stays increased longer after myocardial damage than cTnI.

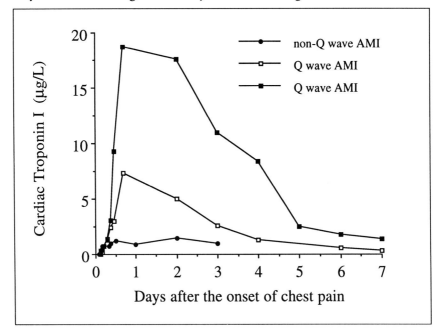

Fig. 5.19. Cardiac troponin I time courses in three patients with acute myocardial infarction without thrombolytic treatment. Abbreviation: acute myocardial infarction (AMI).

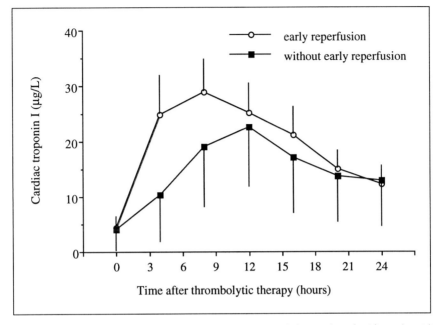

Fig. 5.20. Cardiac troponin I time courses in patients with (n = 15) and without (n = 7) early reperfusion of the infarct-related coronary artery.

Risk stratification in patients with acute coronary syndromes

In healthy individuals circulating cTnI levels are extremely low (below or close to the analytical sensitivity of cTnI assays), which contributes to its high diagnostic sensitivity for detection of even very small events of cardiomyocyte injury.[105] Similar to cTnT, increased cTnI concentrations in serum are found in about 30% of patients with unstable angina Braunwald severity class III (see Fig. 5.21).[105,137] These increases in markers predict a higher cardiac event rate during hospitalization and the subsequent months than in patients without elevated cTnI concentrations. Comparable large studies to cTnT on the prognostic significance of cTnI increase in patients with unstable angina are not yet available, but first results on cTnI[137] are promising and it is very likely that cTnI is comparable with cTnT. Nonetheless, according to currently available data on the risk stratification in patients with unstable angina using troponin measurement cTnT has to be recommended, because more and larger studies have been published on cTnT so far.

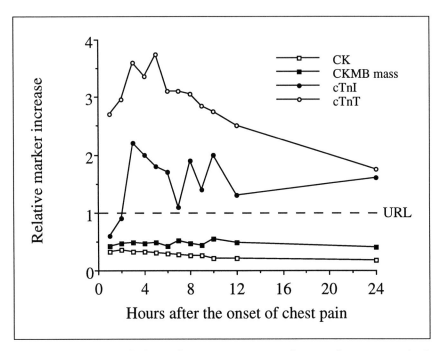

Fig. 5.21. Time course of relative plasma concentrations of creatine kinase activity (CK), CKMB mass, cardiac troponin I and troponin T in a patient with unstable angina pectoris and transient ST-T alterations (Braunwald class III). Relative marker protein increases are given as multiples of each upper reference limit, indicated by the broken line. Abbreviations: creatine kinase (CK), cardiac troponin I (cTnI), cardiac troponin T (cTnT), upper reference limit (URL).

cTnI concentrations after invasive-cardiological procedures

Percutaneous transluminal coronary angioplasty (PTCA), coronary rotational ablation, directional coronary atherectomy (DCA), and related procedures

Similar to cTnT, cTnI is a useful marker to assess myocardial damage after these interventions. In uncomplicated PTCA patients, cTnI does not increase in serum over a baseline measure (see Fig. 5.22).[138] However, angiographically visible occlusion of smaller side-branches next to the site of the dilated stenosis, although symptomless, may lead to a slight increase in cTnI. In these patients and other patients with minor complications (prolonged chest pain, ECG documented episodes of myocardial ischemia) which do not fulfill standard WHO AMI criteria cTnI concentrations after PTCA

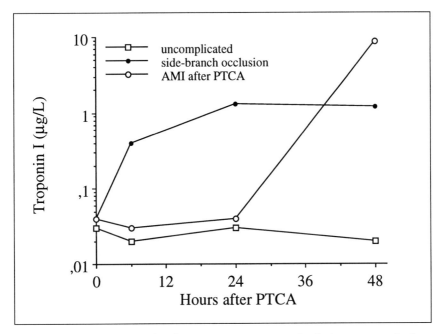

Fig. 5.22. Cardiac troponin I after elective percutaneous transluminal coronary angioplasty (PTCA). Abbreviation: Acute Myocardial Infarction (AMI)

usually stay <1.5 µg/l depending on baseline values within the reference interval. Reocclusion of a successfully dilated stenosis causes a marked rise in cTnI similar to other AMI patients (see Fig. 5.22).

Defibrillation threshold tests during implantation of intracardiac defibrillators

Similar to cTnT, increases in cTnI may be found after this intervention. cTnI release correlated with the duration of fibrillation.

Radiofrequency catheter ablation therapy

After such interventions all myocardial proteins including cTnI frequently increase in blood. There is a relation between increase in markers and the radiofrequency cumulated power and application time.

Diagnosis of perioperative myocardial infarction (PMI)

Diagnosis of perioperative myocardial infarction in noncardiac surgery:

The most important advantage of cTnI is its cardiac-specificity. Thus, cTnI measurements are especially helpful in the assessment of patients with myocardial ischemia and skeletal muscle injury, e.g., after surgery. cTnI was found to be a sensitive and specific method for diagnosis of PMI.[139] cTnI correlated more closely with the appearance of new abnormalities in segmental-wall motion on the postoperative echocardiogram than CKMB and avoids the high incidence of false positive diagnoses associated with the use of CKMB as a diagnostic marker.

Diagnosis of perioperative myocardial infarction (PMI) in coronary artery bypass grafting (CABG) surgery:

As for other cardiac enzymes and proteins after CABG, general reference limits of cTnI are not valid as there is inevitable cardiac tissue damage (e.g., by right atriotomy for cannulation, cardioplegic cardiac arrest, or intermittent aortic cross-clamping)

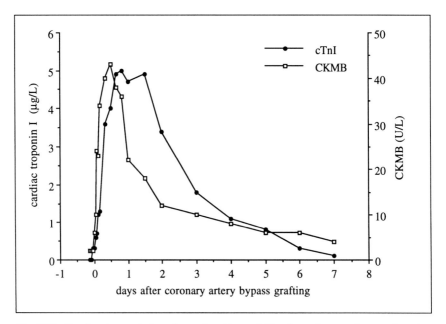

Fig. 5.23. Cardiac troponin I and creatine kinase MB release in a patient undergoing elective coronary artery bypass grafting with non-Q wave perioperative myocardial infarction.

occurring during the surgical procedure (see troponin T). After elective CABG, cTnI peaks >3.7 µg/L and concentrations >3.1 µg/L at 12 hours or >2.5 µg/L at 24 hours indicate PMI.[140] In PMI, cTnI concentrations start increasing with aortic unclamping, peak on or about the 1st postoperative day and remain increased until at least the 5th day after CABG surgery (see Fig. 5.23). cTnI in patients without PMI also significantly increases after reperfusion over values seen before bypass and stays increased for several days (see Fig. 5.24). Peak values occur on average 8 hours after aortic unclamping and usually do not exceed 2.5 µg/L in completely uneventful patients. In patients with aortic valve replacement, cTnI release correlates with aortic cross-clamping time.[141] After CABG surgery there is a third group of patients with minor perioperative myocardial damage.[140] cTnI peaks in these patients are >2.5 µg/L and higher than in completely uneventful patients. However, these patients do not meet the standard criteria of PMI. Nonspecific ECG changes, need for inotropic support of the heart during or after weaning from cardiopulmonary bypass, and transient wall motion abnormalities in echocardiography are frequent in those patients. In summary, cTnI reliably identifies perioperative

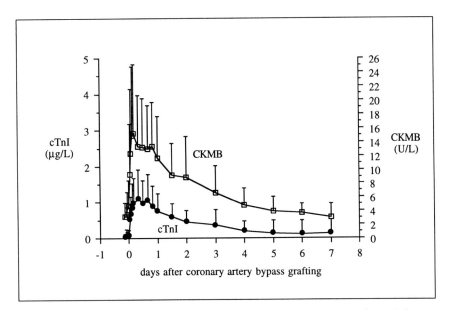

Fig. 5.24. Cardiac troponin I and creatine kinase MB release in uncomplicated elective coronary artery bypass grafting. Data given as mean + SD of 22 patients.

infarction during CABG and is superior to CKMB activity, especially in diagnosing minor perioperative myocardial damage. However, it must be stressed that different discriminator values from that above given may be valid depending on the assay used, because the currently commercially available cTnI assays are not standardized yet (1996 at the time when this manuscript was written). cTnI is also useful in assessing the effectiveness of various cardioprotective measures.

Separate postsurgical cTnI reference intervals have to be evaluated for other cardiac surgical procedures, especially if they include cardiotomy, e.g., mitral valve surgery and CABG during the same operation. For all other cardiac surgical procedures PMI is fortunately a rare complication. If cardiac surgery includes cardiotomy also cTnI is not useful for PMI diagnosis in these patients.

Nonischemic myocardial damage

Myocarditis

Acute myocarditis
A highly sensitive and specific marker, such as cTnI, is needed to accurately diagnose the limited myocardial damage occurring in acute myocarditis. In mice with autoimmune myocarditis cTnI was reported to be a sensitive marker for the presence of disease. cTnI was elevated particularly in histologically diffuse disease.[142] Increased cTnI concentrations were also found in patients with confirmed myocarditis.[142] Again elevations of cTnI when present in patients suggest diffuse disease. Elevations are uncommon with focal myocarditis. The available data suggest that cTnI is a more sensitive and specific parameter than CK and CKMB for detection of myocardial damage in acute myocarditis.

Chronic myocarditis in patients with cardiomyopathies
Similar to cTnT, slightly to moderately increased cTnI can be detected in blood samples from a subgroup of patients with dilated cardiomyopathy, particularly in patients with a poor left ventricular function. This is probably explained by the progressive destruction of cardiomyocytes and may indicate a worse prognosis compared with patients without detectable cTnI.

Heart transplantation

After orthotopic heart transplantation in men, cTnI moderately increases. cTnI returns within the reference interval earlier (within 2-3 weeks) than cTnT. Therefore, cTnI may be more suitable to detect rejection than cTnT, because less frequent blood sampling is necessary to recognize a new increase in cTnI. However, cTnI concentrations cannot predict rejection episodes, because as with all other intramyocardial proteins it only increases in serum when myocardial damage has already occurred.

Similar to cTnT, cTnI can also be used to assess the heart in a potential heart transplant donor.[143] Biochemical evaluation of donor heart damage by measurement of cTnI predicts the response of the heart after transplantation in recipients (see troponin T).

Blunt cardiac trauma

As cTnI measurements are particularly useful in the assessment of cardiac injury in the presence of skeletal muscle damage, it is expected that cTnI more accurately diagnoses heart contusion than CK or LDH isoenzymes, which should facilitate the diagnosis and management of such patients. In fact, it could be demonstrated that serial cTnI measurements are a valuable aid in the diagnosis of blunt cardiac trauma avoiding the numerous false positive CKMB results seen in trauma patients (see figure 5.25).[105,144] However, similar to cTnT, it remains to be demonstrated if patients with increase in cTnI have a worse prognosis than patients without. In contrast to the patients with isolated chest trauma the diagnosis of heart contusion, apart from the obvious, easily clinically diagnosed cases, may be of little prognostic relevance in the multiply injured patient compared with other injuries and their complications.

Diagnostic specificity of cTnI

As the diagnostic sensitivities of cTnI and cTnT are at least as high for the clinical detection of cardiac injury as of CKMB mass, and the sensitivities of cTnI and cTnT are roughly equivalent, current discussions about cardiac markers are highly focused on the cardiac specificity of these proteins, in particular on the specificities of cTnI and cTnT. The selection of monoclonal antibodies directed against the cardiac-specific region of the cTnI molecule

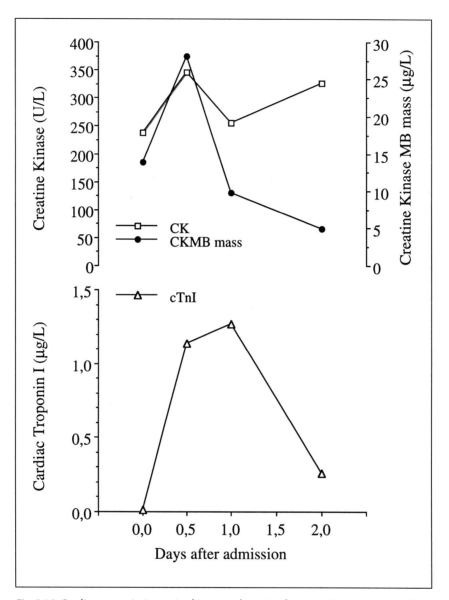

Fig. 5.25. Cardiac troponin I, creatine kinase and creatine kinase MB mass concentrations in a multiple injury patient with heart contusion. Despite an increase in CKMB mass, the CKMB/CK index was negative in all samples. Abbreviation: creatine kinase (CK), cardiac troponin I (cTnI).

led to highly specific antibodies which do not crossreact with skeletal muscle TnI isoforms. On this basis and on the biochemical basis of cTnI, measurement of cTnI in serum can be considered as extraordinarily specific for the detection of myocyte injury in humans.

Increased cTnI is not detectable in the circulation of multiply traumatized patients or athletes after strenuous exercise, in patients with acute or chronic skeletal muscle disease, in renal failure cases, or in patients with elevated CKMB unless concomitant myocardial injury has occurred (see Table 5.5).[105,145,146] Elevations of cTnI correlate closely with evidence for myocardial injury demonstrated by echocardiography. cTnI is suitable to biochemically assess myocardial injury in critically ill patients and patients with multiple organ failure in which clinical histories often are unreliable, ECG

Table 5.5. Specificity of cardiac troponin I in patients with concomitant skeletal muscle damage

	CK peak* (U/L; 37°C)	CKMB mass peak* (μg/L)	CKMB/CK (37°C) >2.5%	cTnI peak (μg/L)
Marathon runners after race (n = 18)	297 (102 – 527)	9.8 (6.2 – 16.5)	in 14 runners	<0.1
Myopathy after eccentric exercise (n = 16)	2144 (400 – 49294)	7.3 (5.1 – 12.2)	in no athlete	<0.1
Duchenne MD (n = 5)	7795 (4653 – 20096)	187.7 (65 – 376.2)	in 1 patient	<0.1
Becker MD (n = 4)	4266 (518 – 9989)	70.9 (4.8 – 200.6)	in 2 patients	<0.1
Multitrauma (n = 17)	1877 (679 – 26231)	22.5 (5.3 – 175.8)	in 2 patients	<0.1
Multitrauma with heart contusion (n = 2)	3110 852	23.4 28.1	no yes	0.22 1.27

* Apart from patients with heart contusion data are given as median and range (in parentheses)
   Abbreviations: muscular dystrophy (MD)
   The upper reference limit of the cardiac troponin I assay used is 0.1 μg/L.

changes are ubiquitous, and elevations of CKMB are difficult to interpret. Thus far, in all published studies elevations of cTnI could be definitively attributed to myocardial damage or myocardial damage was the obvious cause of cTnI increase.

Clinical use of cTnI—Summary

cTnI is a highly sensitive and specific marker for myocardial damage and appears to be ideally suited for its diagnosis in complex clinical situations with concomitant skeletal muscle injury. The clinical indications for cTnI measurement are the same as for cTnT (see troponin T). However, for monitoring of thrombolytic therapy or risk stratification in patients with unstable angina fewer data are currently available for the use of cTnI than for cTnT. On the other hand, cTnI may be more suitable for detecting rejection episodes in heart transplant recipients (see above), and cTnI is currently the marker of choice for detecting or excluding biochemically myocardial injury in patients with chronic myopathies, renal diseases, or multiple organ failure.

MYOSIN HEAVY CHAINS (MHC)

The MHC in human myocardium consist of two isoforms, α and β, both of which are present in ventricles and atria. They are products of two different genes and represent high and low ATPase activity.[81] In human ventricles β-type MHC is almost the exclusive form present at all ages (approximately 90%), and no marked difference is found during hypertrophy.[81] Cardiac β-type MHC is identical to slow-twitch skeletal MHC and is coexpressed in slow-twitch skeletal muscle fibers.[147] Human atrial muscle essentially contains α-type MHC. Chronic hemodynamic overload induces a transition from α- to β-type MHC, i.e., from an atrial to a ventricular isoform.[81] α-type MHC may provide a more specific marker of myocardial damage. The expression of this MHC isoform has been thought to be exclusive to the myocardium. However, cardiac α-type MHC has been found in human masticatory muscles (skeletal muscles originating from the cranial part of the embryo).[148] Moreover, β-type MHC predominates (90%) also in normal human left ventricular myocardium,[149] which may limit the diagnostic sensitivity of α-type MHC.

We found no evidence for a soluble MHC pool in the sarcoplasma (unpublished results), and all MHC of muscle fibers appears to be structurally bound. Therefore, this protein is expected to specifically indicate myocardial necrosis, because for its release more severe damage is required, i.e., an increased permeability of the sarcolemma for macromolecules together with a degradation or dissociation of the thick filaments of the contractile apparatus. For the release of cytoplasmatic proteins, such as myoglobin and CK, in principal only an altered plasma membrane permeability is necessary.

As a consequence of its tissue distribution, all MHC assays described in the literature so far,[150,151] considerably cross-reacted with MHC from skeletal muscle and are, therefore, not superior to CKMB or LDH-1 with respect to specificity. Apart from myocardial infarction, at present, no data on MHC release in other cardiac diseases are available.

MHC release kinetics in AMI patients

MHC is a molecule of large size and low solubility without a soluble precursor pool in sarcoplasma. It has been shown that rather than the intact MHC molecule, it is soluble fragments that are detected in serum after AMI.[151] Myosin is efficiently proteolyzed into fragments as soon as it is liberated from the myocyte.[150] MHC fragments appear about 1-3 days in the circulation and are detectable to about 10 days after the onset of AMI.[136,150-153] This delay in plasma release is longer than for any other cytosolic or contractile protein so far assayed. MHC may be the most suitable marker to quantify the extent of myocardial necrosis after infarction.[152] This delayed appearance of MHC in the bloodstream precludes its use in the early phase of AMI and restricts MHC measurements for late AMI diagnosis or the assessment of infarct size. The time course is monophasic and MHC peaks several days (5-7) after the onset of AMI (see Fig. 5.26). The average maximal MHC peak value is 40 times greater the average MHC concentration in a normal population.[150] MHC and MLC peak values correlated closely.[136,153] MHC release is slightly accelerated by successful thrombolytic treatment. In patients with reperfusion, peak values occur on an average 1 day earlier and are like cumulative MHC release values significantly lower in patients with reperfusion[152,153] (see also Fig. 5.27).

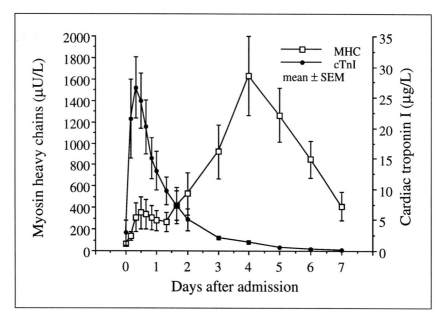

Fig. 5.26. Myosin heavy chain (MHC) and cardiac troponin I (cTnI) time courses after myocardial infarction. Data given as mean ± SEM of 18 patients.

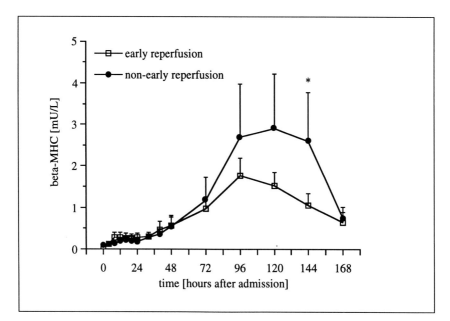

Fig. 5.27. Influence of early reperfusion on cardiac β-type myosin heavy chain release. Data given as mean + standard error of the mean (SEM). Asterisk indicates significant difference between patient groups (early reperfusion: n = 16; without early reperfusion: n = 7).

Although cTnI, cTnT, and β-type MHC are all constituents of the contractile apparatus of muscle fibers, the differences in concentration time courses after AMI are striking. There is no evidence for the existence of a soluble cytosolic MHC pool in cardiomyocytes. Because of the central location of MHC in the thick filament, it is more resistant to proteolysis,[150] which may account for the differences observed in troponin and β-type MHC time courses after AMI.

MHC to quantify the extent of myocardial necrosis

Thrombolytic therapy does not qualitatively upset MHC kinetics. MHC release is monophasic. From a practical point of view, only a few serial (daily) determinations of serum MHC concentrations are enough to estimate infarct size. The maximal MHC concentrations are strongly correlated with cumulative MHC release (r = 0.85).[152] In an experimental canine myocardial infarction model, the necrosed myocardial mass correlated very closely with cumulative MHC release (r = 0.88).[152] In AMI patients, cumulative CK, CKMB, LDH and MHC release were correlated closely. Cumulative MHC release also correlated closely (r = 0.77) with thallium-201 estimates of myocardial scar.[152] MHC release was of prognostic value in 1 year follow-up of AMI patients. However, it remains to be seen in a larger AMI patient series, whether cumulative MHC release correlates considerably closer with other independent estimates of myocardial scar (e.g., myocardial scintigraphy, positron emission tomography, magnetic resonance imaging) than cumulative cTnT, cTnI, CKMB, or LDH-1 release.

MHC in cardiac surgery

MHC is a sensitive indicator of myocardial necrosis after cardiac operation.[154] After CABG surgery, MHC concentrations increase also in uncomplicated patients similar to all other markers (see troponin T, troponin I). MHC starts to increase from postoperative day 3 and reaches peak values on day 7, and then decreases regularly. Peak MHC values in patients with PMI after CABG were significantly higher than in patients without (see Fig. 5.28). MHC only allows late diagnosis of myocardial damage.

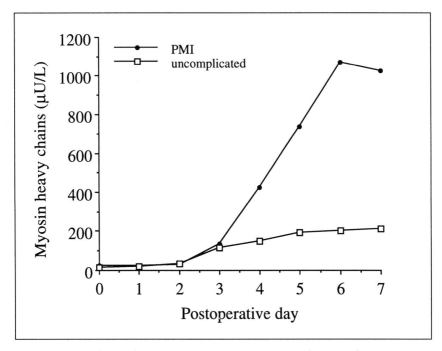

Fig. 5.28. Myosin heavy chain time courses in two patients undergoing elective coronary artery bypass grafting, one without and one with perioperative non-Q wave myocardial infarction. Abbreviation: Perioperative Myocardial Infarction (PMI)

Clinical use of MHC—Summary

MHC is not a heart-specific marker. Currently there are no clinical settings in which MHC is clearly superior to the other markers. Even in the quantification of infarct size in AMI patients its superiority over the other markers remains to be demonstrated. MHC will probably gain no importance for routine use in hospital laboratories. Its application will probably be restricted to scientific investigations.

MYOSIN LIGHT CHAINS (MLC)

The slow-twitch skeletal muscle MLC-1 and MLC-2 are identical with the cardiac MLC-1 and MLC-2.[79,80,155] In the mouse and rat both slow skeletal MLC-1 and cardiac MLC-1 are encoded by a single gene.[79] Amino acid sequence analyses strongly indicate the identity of slow skeletal MLC-2 and cardiac MLC-2 in rabbit and chicken.[80] In addition, there is very high amino acid sequence homology among MLCs. A minor fraction of MLC (approximately 1% of the total MLC content) exists as a soluble cytoplasmatic precursor pool for myosin synthesis.[156,157] The cytosolic pool of cTnT is approximately 50 times larger compared with MLC-1.[90]

Radioimmunoassays for the detection of cardiac MLC were the first assays of contractile proteins to be described in the literature.[158,159] At that time, cardiac MLC appeared to be proteins unique to myocardium. During subsequent years, however, it turned out that in various animals cardiac MLC-1 and MLC-2 are coexpressed in slow skeletal muscle fibers (see above), which is probably also true in men. MLC assays showed varying cross-reactivity with MLC isolated from skeletal muscle. However, several investigators are still studying the possibility of a unique cardiac MLC-1 isoform that is not expressed in other muscle types. Up to now, researchers failed to demonstrate the superiority of their cardiac MLC assays over CKMB and LDH-1 determinations with respect to diagnostic specificity in large clinical evaluations. MLC release in ischemic myocardial damage has been studied extensively.

Acute myocardial infarction

Both, cardiac MLC-1 and MLC-2, appear as early as CK and rise within hours (4-12) after the onset of the attack. In most patients, MLC can be detected in serum within 6 hours after the onset of infarct-related symptoms. For the first 48 hours, the sensitivity of MLC is equal to CKMB activity. cTnI and cTnT increase earlier than MLC (see Fig. 5.29).[136,153] However, MLC-1 and MLC-2 peak about day 4 and remain elevated for 1-2 weeks despite a serum half-life of approximately 2 hours.[136,153,157-160] Two sub-trends of MLC-1 release were discerned: in the majority of patients MLC-1 release is monophasic, in some patients, however, release is biphasic. MLC-1 levels increase and then decrease to normal levels 1-2 days after the initial rise. Subsequently, MLC-1 becomes elevated again for the next 5-9 days after the onset of the attack.[161] MLC and MHC peaks correlate closely.[153] The initial increase in serum MLC is probably from the soluble MLC pool in the myocyte while prolonged increase in MLC is from proteolytic degradation or pH dissociation of myosin liberating the myofilaments.[161] The early appearance of MLC as well as their persistence make possible a diagnosis in the acute phase of AMI and in the evaluation of patients who present late in the course of the disease.

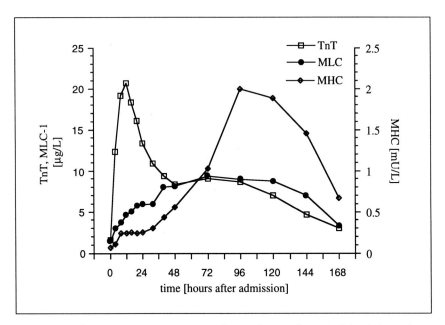

Fig. 5.29. Cardiac troponin T, β-type myosin heavy chain and myosin light chain-1 release after acute myocardial infarction. Curves represent the mean values of the 23 patients investigated. Abbreviations: Troponin T (TnT), myosin light chain (MLC), myosin heavy chain (MHC).

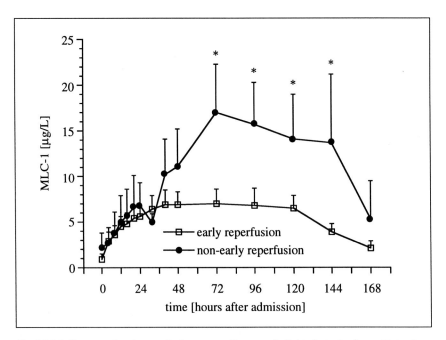

Fig. 5.30. Influence of early reperfusion on cardiac myosin light chain-1 release. Data given as mean + standard error of the mean (SEM). Asterisks indicate significant difference between patient groups (early reperfusion: n = 16; without early reperfusion: n = 7).

MLC release in thrombolytic treatment

Release of MLC is not significantly changed by recanalization of the infarct-related artery compared with that in nonreperfused myocardial infarction (see Fig. 5.30) and the time to peak value of MLC is almost independent of early infarct perfusion.[153,162] Peak appearance time is about 4 days regardless of reperfusion.[163] Peak levels of MLC are lower in AMI patients with early reperfusion (see Fig. 5.30) and are closely related to the left ventricular ejection fraction regardless of the presence of coronary reperfusion.[163]

MLC release is closely related to infarct size

Close linear correlations between MLC-2 serum concentrations and the extent of myocardial necrosis have been shown in experimental animals. Of all biochemical markers tested, infarct size in dogs correlated most closely with MLC-2 release.[164] In AMI patients, the severity of infarction and mortality are positively and the left ventricular ejection fraction inversely correlated with MLC cumulative appearance.[160] A close correlation was found between the cumulative appearance of MLC and their peak values. Peak concentrations of MLC correlate well with scintigraphic estimates of myocardial scar.[165,166]

MLC in coronary artery bypass grafting

MLC is a sensitive indicator of myocardial necrosis after cardiac surgery.[167] After CABG surgery, MLC concentrations increase also in uncomplicated patients similar to all other markers (see troponin T, troponin I). In patients without PMI, MLC reach a first peak at 6 hours after aortic declamping, and after falling slightly, they increase again to reach the second and maximum peak on day 3. In PMI, MLC gradually increase and peak on postoperative day 3. Peak MLC values and values on day 1-5 in patients with PMI after CABG were significantly higher than in patients without.[167] MLC could discriminate both groups from the first postoperative day. cTnT could identify extensive myocardial damage earlier than MLC-1.[167]

MLC in patients with angina pectoris at rest

Similar to cTnT, in about 30% of patients with acute angina at rest increased serum concentrations of MLC are found in serial blood samples.[20] Increase in MLC is an independent risk factor for the development of cardiac events during the subsequent months.[20] The presence of MLC correlated with signs of ischemia in ECG. Elevated marker protein concentrations were found only in patients with coronary artery stenosis ≥75% of at least one major coronary artery. The detection of MLC in serum indicates ischemic damage of small myocardial areas and identifies a subgroup of patients with angina at rest having severe coronary artery disease. These patients are at risk to develop AMI and other cardiac events including cardiac death.

MLC in other diseases

Cardiac MLC is not a heart-specific marker. Increased serum levels of human cardiac MLC-1 compared with normal controls have been reported in patients with renal failure.[168] Increased serum cardiac MLC-1 has also been described in patients with Duchenne muscular dystrophy.[169] The levels of MLC-1 have obvious positive correlation with CK and myoglobin and have a close relationship with the functional disturbances of skeletal muscles, especially disturbances of pulmonary ventilation.

Clinical use of MLC—Summary

According to current knowledge MLC is not a heart-specific marker. Currently there are no clinical settings in which MLC is clearly superior to the other markers, in particular cTnI and cTnT. Even in the quantification of infarct size in AMI patients MLC was not superior to cTnT.[166] MLC measurement will probably gain no importance for routine use in hospital laboratories. Based on current information cTnI and cTnT offer the most exciting potential as markers of myocardial damage.

GLYCOGEN PHOSPHORYLASE ISOENZYME BB

In the final analysis myoglobin, CKMB mass, CK isoforms, and troponins are not sufficiently sensitive within the first 3-4 hours after the onset of AMI, and the diagnostic performance of the ECG is clearly superior to that of biochemical markers during this time interval.[4,12-14,54,170] However, up to 50% of chest pain patients may have nondiagnostic ECGs at hospital admission.[13,170] Laboratory parameters are cheaper, easier to perform and to interpret for the nonspecialist than other alternative diagnostic methods (e.g., echocardiography, myocardial scintigraphy). Consequently the search is still going on for more rapidly detectable and more sensitive markers which should start to be released in the phase of reversible ischemic myocardial damage. In this respect, glycogen phosphorylase isoenzyme BB (GPBB) based on its metabolic function and on first clinical results is a very promising enzyme for the early laboratory detection of ischemic myocardial injury.

BIOCHEMISTRY

Glycogen phosphorylase (GP) is one of the best-studied enzymes in biochemistry. It is a glycolytic enzyme which plays an essential role in the regulation of carbohydrate metabolism by mobilization of glycogen.[171] It catalyzes the first step in glycogenolysis in which glycogen is converted to glucose-1-phosphate, utilizing inorganic phosphate. The physiological role of muscle phosphorylase is to provide the fuel for the energy supply required for muscle contraction. Its activity is allosterically regulated by the binding of AMP and phosphorylation. Phosphorylase kinase converts GP b into its more active form GP a. Phosphorylase exists in the cardiomyocyte in association with glycogen and the sarcoplasmatic reticulum and forms a macromolecular complex (sarcoplasmatic reticulum glycogenolysis complex).[172,173] The degree of association of GP with this complex depends essentially on the metabolic state of the myocardium (see Fig. 5.31). With the onset of tissue hypoxia, when glycogen is broken down and disappears, glycogen phosphorylase is converted from a particulate into a soluble form, and the enzyme becomes free to move around in the cytoplasma.[172-174]

GP exists as a dimer under normal physiological conditions. The dimer is composed of two identical subunits. At least three GP isoenzymes are found in human tissues that are named after the tissue in which they are preferentially expressed, GPLL (liver), GPMM (muscle), and GPBB (brain).[171] The three isoenzymes can be distinguished by functional and immunological properties. They are encoded by three distinct genes. The genes of the three human GP isoenzymes have been cloned and sequenced.[175] The proteins predicted by the cDNA sequences are 846 (LL), 842 (MM) and 862 (BB) amino acids long. Amino acids 1-830 match and differences are mainly found at the C-terminus, which is the catalytic domain of the protein. In pairwise sequence comparison the brain-type protein is 80% identical to the liver type and 83%

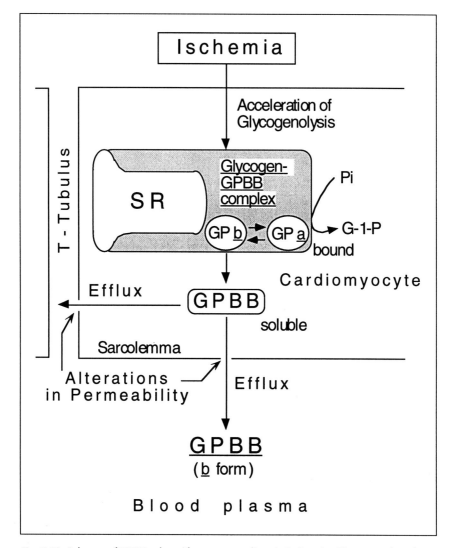

Fig. 5.31. Scheme of GPBB release from myocardium in ischemia. Glycogen phosphorylase (GP) together with glycogen are tightly associated with the vesicles of sarcoplasmatic
reticulum (SR) under normal conditions. A release of GPBB, the main isoform in the
myocardium, essentially depends on the degradation of glycogen, which is catalyzed by
GP a (the phosphorylated, active form of the isoenzyme) and by GP b (nonphosphorylated,
AMP-dependent form). Ischemia is known to favor the conversion of bound GP b into GP
a and thereby accelerating glycogen breakdown, which seems to be the ultimate
prerequisite for getting GP into a soluble form. An efflux of GPBB into the extracellular fluid
may only follow if ischemia-induced structural alterations in the cell membrane are
manifested. Pi: inorganic phosphate; G-1-P: glucose-1-phosphate. For more details see
text. Adapted from Ref. 186.

identical to the muscle type. GPBB has 21 and 16 additional amino acid residues on its C-terminal portion that are not present on the MM and LL isoenzymes, respectively.

Adult human skeletal muscle contains only one isoenzyme, GPMM. GPLL is the predominant isoenzyme in human liver and all other human tissues except for heart, skeletal muscle and brain. The isoenzyme BB is the predominant isoenzyme of human brain. Its molecular weight as a monomer is approximately 94 kDa. In the human heart the isoenzymes BB and MM are found, but GPBB is the predominant isoenzyme in myocardium as well. By far the highest concentrations of GPBB were found in human brain and heart. The tissue concentrations of GPBB in heart and brain are comparable.[176] Although immunoblot, electrophoresis, and northern blot data are partly conflicting,[171,175-178] there is evidence that GPBB isoenzyme might not be restricted to brain and heart in humans. Much lower GPBB concentrations have been reported for example in leukocytes, platelets, spleen, kidney, bladder, testis, digestive tract and aorta. However, in all these tissues the isoenzyme LL is by far the predominant GP isoenzyme. In addition, GPBB is expressed in fetal rat skeletal muscle.[171] Whether GPBB is expressed in human fetal skeletal muscle or whether GPBB may be reexpressed, similar to CKMB and LDH isoenzyme 1, in human regenerating adult skeletal muscle, such as in Duchenne muscular dystrophy, is not yet sufficiently investigated.

PATHOPHYSIOLOGY: MYOCARDIAL OXYGEN DEFICIENCY AND GPBB RELEASE

As outlined above the sarcoplasmic reticulum-glycogenolysis complex represents a functionally coupled association (see Fig. 5.31). There is a close relationship between glycogenolysis and excitation and contraction coupling and/or β-adrenergic stimulation of the myocardium. During acute ischemia a sympathetic activation of the myocardium is followed by a transient rise in cardiac cAMP levels and by an activation of GP due to a conversion of the nonphosphorylated b form into phosphorylase a by phosphorylase kinase.[179] Concomitantly the rate of glycogenolysis was found to be accelerated. Kinetic properties of GPBB allow furthermore a glycogen breakdown catalyzed by the b form. An ischemia-induced rise in the levels of intracellular orthophosphate and AMP in myocardium may therefore induce a second, long-lasting acceleration of glycogenolysis under these conditions. In fact, cardiac glycogen breakdown was found to be continued during postischemic reperfusion when the a form of GP was decreased to pre-ischemic control levels but the orthophosphate level was still high.[180] In experimental studies as well as in patients with AMI the released GPBB was exclusively found in the b form.[181,182] Thus it is suggested that the activity of GPBB (form b) catalyzes the prolonged degradation of glycogen in the sarcoplasmatic reticulum-glycogenolysis complex in the ischemic area of the myocardium.[179]

In conscious dogs a rapid release of GPBB was measured in the cardiac lymph after a transient ligation of a coronary artery not longer than 10 minutes, which did not lead to histological signs of myocardial necrosis.[181] An efflux of GP from the myocar-

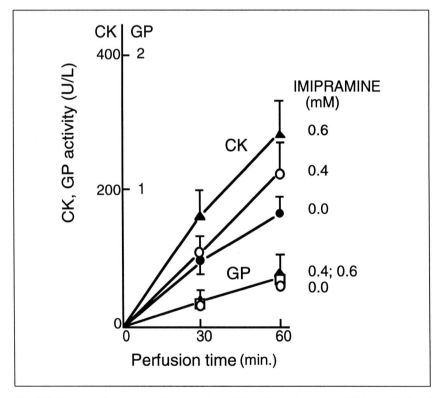

Fig. 5.32. Release of glycogen phosphorylase (GP) and creatine kinase (CK) from isolated perfused rabbit hearts. The effect of 0.4 and 0.6 mM imipramine were only studied with nonbeating hearts at 24 °C. 0.0 mM imipramine represents the controls. These experimental results are published in Krause et al.[184]

dium after hypoxia or substrate depletion has been observed earlier in the isolated perfused rat and rabbit heart.[183,184] The GP release in these experiments correlated with the remaining myocardial glycogen content.[184] In this Langendorff model of the isolated perfused rabbit heart the addition of imipramine under aerobic conditions to a cardioplegic perfusion solution only caused a release of CK, but not of GP (see Fig. 5.32).[184] The myocardial glycogen content remained unaffected as well. Imipramine causes in a certain concentration range a selective increase in the plasma membrane permeability without myocardial hypoxia. On the other hand, the stimulation of glycogenolysis by high doses of epinephrine did not cause a decrease in myocardial GP activity, although the glycogen content of the tissue was greatly diminished by the added epinephrine.[183] These experimental results allow the conclusion that the release of GPBB requires both a burst in glycogenolysis and a concomitantly increased plasma membrane permeability as it is known for ischemically injured cardiomyocytes.

Given its molecular mass the early release of GPBB raises questions on the mechanisms of its release from ischemic myocardium. An essential part of an explanation may be its key role in the energy metabolism of ischemic myocardium. When glycogen is broken down and disappears, GPBB becomes free to move from the perisarcoplasmatic reticulum compartment directly into the extracellular fluid, if cell membrane permeability is simultaneously increased, which is usually the case in ischemia. A high GPBB concentration gradient, which immediately is formed in the compartment of the sarcoplasmatic reticulum glycogenolytic complex, may be the reason for the high efflux rate of this enzyme. In contrast to other cytosolic proteins, this gradient may be at least partly realized via T-tubuli and may contribute to the efflux of GPBB (see Fig. 5.31).

In summary, the ischemia-sensitive glycogen degradation, which is regulated by Ca^{2+}, metabolic intermediates and catecholamines, seems to be a crucial prerequisite for the efflux of GPBB. This outlines the specific sensitivity of this enzyme marker to transient imbalances in heart energy metabolism as it is the case during angina pectoris attacks and/or in the infarcting myocardium. Therefore, this enzyme is a promising analyte for the detection of ischemic myocardial injury.

First Clinical Results

Acute myocardial infarction

There were distinct differences in sensitivities of GPBB in comparison to myoglobin, CKMB mass, CK and cTnT within the first 2-3 hours after AMI onset,[185,186] and GPBB was the most sensitive parameter during the first 4 hours after AMI onset. In the majority of AMI patients GPBB increased between 1 and 4 hours after the onset of chest pain (see Fig. 5.33). Therefore, GPBB may be a very important marker for the early diagnosis of AMI. GPBB usually peaks before CK, CKMB or cTnT and returns within the reference interval within 1-2 days after AMI onset.[186] Similar to soluble markers, such as myoglobin and CKMB, we could demonstrate that GPBB time courses in AMI patients are markedly influenced by the occurrence of early reperfusion of the infarct-related coronary artery.[186] The well-established so-called "wash out" phenomenon after successful thrombolysis leads to a more rapid increase in GPBB, and earlier and higher peak values

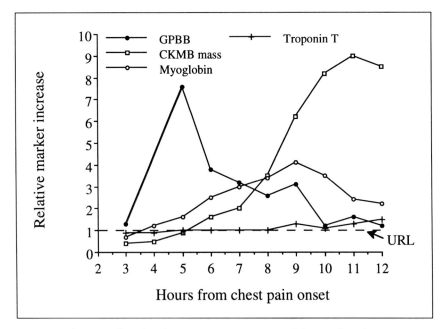

Fig. 5.33. Glycogen phosphorylase BB, CKMB mass, myoglobin, and cardiac troponin T time courses in a patient with a small non-Q wave myocardial infarction. Data are given as x-fold increase of the upper reference limit (URL).

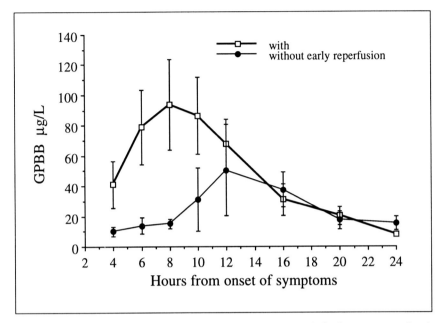

Fig. 5.34. Glycogen phosphorylase BB in patients with myocardial infarction treated with thrombolytic agents. Patients were grouped according to early reperfusion of the infarct-related coronary artery. Data given as mean ± SEM (early reperfusion: n = 9; without early reperfusion: n = 5).

(see Fig. 5.34). Therefore, GPBB may be useful, alongside with other soluble myocardial proteins, to assess noninvasively the effectiveness of thrombolytic therapy. However, decision limits to detect successful, and, what is clinically more important, failed reperfusion, remain to be established in an acutely performed coronary angiography controlled study.

Unstable angina pectoris

The application of GPBB is not restricted to conventional myocardial infarction. An early release of GPBB was demonstrated in patients with Braunwald class III unstable angina who showed ST-T alterations at rest. Only GPBB was increased above the upper reference limit in the majority of these patients at hospital admission (see Fig. 5.35).[187] Whether the early GPBB release in these patients is due to minimal necrosis of myocardial tissue or severe reversible ischemic injury is currently not known. As underlined by the receiver-operating characteristic (ROC) curve and

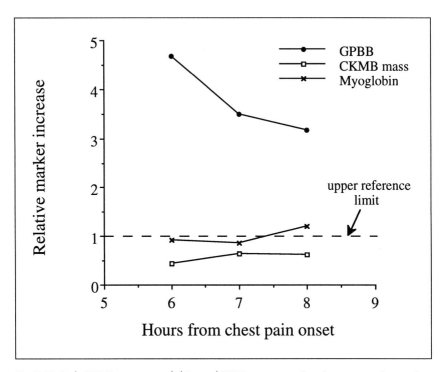

Fig. 5.35. Early CKMB mass, myoglobin, and GPBB concentration time courses in a patient with unstable angina who was admitted to the coronary care unit for ruling out myocardial infarction.

ROC area calculations of GPBB and comparison with those of CK, CKMB mass, myoglobin, and cTnT,[186] GPBB showed the best diagnostic performance of all markers tested to detect acute ischemic coronary syndromes (AMI or severe unstable angina at rest with transient ST-T alterations) on hospital admission. GPBB plasma concentrations in patients with stable angina resembled those of healthy individuals or patients without angina.[186]

Coronary artery bypass grafting (CABG)

GPBB is also a sensitive marker for the detection of perioperative myocardial ischemia and infarction in patients undergoing CABG.[188] In uncomplicated patients GPBB peaks within 4 hours after aortic unclamping and returns to baseline values within 20 hours. GPBB release correlates with aortic crossclamping time, which reflects the duration of myocardial hypoxia during cardioplegic cardiac arrest. GPBB time courses of patients with perioperative myocardial infarction (PMI) differ markedly in time to peak values (peaks occur later) and peak concentrations (>50 µg/L) from uneventful patients. However also patients with severe episodes of perioperative myocardial ischemia which do not fulfill standard PMI criteria show markedly elevated GPBB concentrations compared with uncomplicated patients. In patients with emergency CABG, GPBB but not CKMB correlated with clinical evidence of myocardial ischemia.[188] In summary, GPBB is a very sensitive marker of perioperative ischemic myocardial injury in CABG patients.

Diagnostic specificity of GPBB

GPBB is not a heart-specific marker and its specificity is limited. However, increases in GPBB are specific for ischemic myocardial injury when damage to the brain and consequent disturbance of the blood-brain barrier can be excluded clinically. According to experimental studies and clinical observations increases in GPBB do not occur in response to therapeutic circumstances in which cardiac work is increased and glycogen might be mobilized, such as after administration of catecholamines and glucagon, so far a concomitant myocardial injury with cell membrane damage is not processed.[183,188] The diagnostic specificity of GPBB for myocardial injury in nontraumatic chest pain patients was in the range of CKMB,[186] which suggests sufficient specificity in clinical practice. Future studies on the diagnostic specificity of GPBB, however, will also have to address the issue in an unselected group of patients including severely traumatized patients with and without head injuries, and patients with liver damage or renal failure. As long as the diagnostic specificity of GPBB for myocardial damage is not fully delineated, a positive GPBB result should be later confirmed, for example by cTnI measurement.

CLINICAL USE OF GPBB—SUMMARY

Although the first hints that blood GP increases above its upper reference limit early after the onset of AMI before CK does were obtained approximately two decades ago when measuring total GP activity with not very sensitive enzymatic assays.[182] The breakthrough was later the development of a sensitive and specific immunoenzymometric assay for the measurement of the isoenzyme GPBB.[186] The challenge still is to develop a rapid assay which is suitable for bedside or "stat" use in the routine laboratory. Of course, these first clinical results have to be confirmed in a larger number of patients, but they allow several important conclusions, and there is no doubt that GPBB is a promising marker for the detection of ischemic myocardial injury. This is probably explained by its function as a key enzyme of glycogenolysis. GPBB was the most sensitive marker for the diagnosis of AMI within 4 hours after the onset of chest pain. GPBB was the only marker which was increased in a considerable proportion of AMI patients within 2-3 hours after the onset of chest pain.[185,186] The application of GPBB is not restricted to conventional AMI. GPBB also increased early in patients with unstable angina and reversible ST-T alterations in the resting ECG at hospital admission.[186,187] Therefore GPBB could be useful for early risk stratification in these patients. GPBB was also a sensitive marker for the detection of perioperative myocardial ischemia and infarction in patients undergoing coronary artery bypass grafting.[188] The diagnostic specificity of GPBB is sufficient for clinical practice. In nontraumatic chest pain patients it was in the range of that of CKMB.[186] Thus, if these first clinical results on GPBB can be confirmed, the future scenario for the laboratory testing for myocardial injury could be the combination of GPBB measurement with a cardiac-specific marker (e.g., cardiac troponin I), which combines absolute cardiac specificity with high early sensitivity for ischemic myocardial damage.

HEART FATTY ACID BINDING PROTEIN (H-FABP)

Another protein which gained increasing interest for the early diagnosis of AMI and acute coronary syndromes is the soluble heart fatty acid binding protein (H-FABP). There are two groups of FABPs, the sarcolemmal FABPs and the cytoplasmatic FABPs. Only the cytoplasmatic FABP was evaluated as a marker for myocardial damage. This small cytoplasmatic protein (15 kDa) is abundant in cardiomyocytes and is assumed to be involved in myocardial lipid homeostasis. It is one of the most abundant cytoplasmatic proteins in the heart (about 15% of all proteins in the cytoplasma; 0.5 mg/g wet weight).

BIOCHEMISTRY: FABP FUNCTIONS IN THE CARDIOMYOCYTE

Fatty acids play an important role in cardiac energy metabolism. 60-90% of the energy necessary for contraction and other

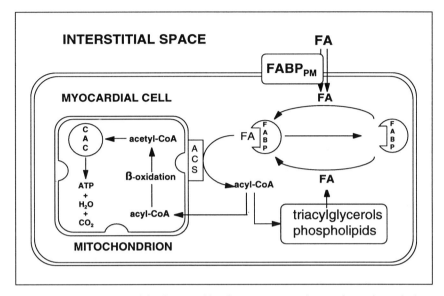

Fig. 5.36. Assumed role of the fatty acid-binding proteins in the uptake and metabolism of long-chain fatty acids (FA) in cardiomyocytes. Fatty acids are either obtained from the plasma albumin-FA complex or by lipoproteinlipase catalyzed hydrolysis of circulating triacyl-glycerols. Abbreviations: Coenzyme A (CoA), acyl-coenzyme A synthase (ACS), citric acid cycle (CAC), plasmalemmal FABP (FABP$_{PM}$), cytoplasmatic FABP (FABP). Adapted from Glatz et al TIJDSCHR NVKC 1993; 18: 144-50.

ATP requiring processes is provided by β-oxidation. The majority of metabolized fatty acids are obtained from the plasma. FABP is involved in the uptake, transport, and metabolism of fatty acids (see Fig. 5.36),[189,190] but its precise role remains to be determined. Besides being an energy substrate, fatty acids are also used in anabolic processes, such as synthesis of triacylglycerols, phospholipids and cholesterol esters. The sarcolemmal FABPs (MW: 40 kDa) are spanning both phospholipid layers and are involved in the cellular uptake of long-chain fatty acids, whereas the soluble cytoplasmatic FABPs are responsible for the intracellular transport of fatty acids. The long-chain fatty acids are poorly soluble in the hydrophilic cytoplasma, and soluble FABP is generally assumed to function as an intracellular counterpart of plasma albumin. Albumin serves as a carrier of fatty acids in the blood stream and interstitial space. FABP facilitates the transport of long-chain fatty acids from the site of entry into the cell (plasma membrane) to the intracellular sites of metabolic conversion (see Fig. 5.36; reviewed in ref. 190).

The Family of Cytoplasmatic FABPs

At least six distinct types of cytoplasmatic FABP are identified and named after the tissue of their first identification, which in general is the tissue of their greatest abundance.[190] The highest FABP contents are found in tissues with high rates of fatty acid handling (intestine, liver, adipose tissue, heart). Each of these tissues has its own soluble FABP type, and each tissue contains at least one FABP type. The amino acid sequence of cytoplasmatic FABPs from different tissues differs. The H-FABP differs in at least 35% of its amino acid composition from the other FABP types, and it was possible to develop specific monoclonal antibodies against H-FABP.[191,192]

Tissue Distribution and Tissue Concentrations of Heart-FABP (H-FABP)

The so-called "heart-FABPs" are not heart-specific. They are also found in considerable amounts in skeletal muscle and kidneys[190] and are, therefore, not a more specific marker for myocardial damage than myoglobin. In an immunohistochemical study staining for H-FABP was frequently observed also in parietal cells of the stomach, the salivary gland, corpus luteum, and Leydig cells of the testis, adipocytes and vascular endothelial cells.[193] But the major sources of false positive plasma concentrations referring to myocardial damage will undoubtedly be skeletal or renal damage.

H-FABP is distributed uniformly in the heart.[194] There are no transmural gradients. Similar to myoglobin and LDH, there is a

Table 5.6. Myoglobin and heart fatty acid binding protein (H-FABP) contents of human heart and skeletal muscle[194]

Tissue	Myoglobin (mg/g wwt)	H-FABP (mg/g wwt)	Myoglobin/ H-FABP
Heart	2.35 ± 0.51	0.52 ± 0.06	4.5 ± 0.8
Skeletal Muscle	3.50 ± 0.50*	0.07 ± 0.03*	20 - 70*

*Strongly dependent on the fiber-type composition of the investigated muscle.
Abbreviations: wet weight (wwt)

negative relation between heart weight and cardiac tissue content of H-FABP. The H-FABP concentrations in human myocardium are higher than cardiac myoglobin concentrations as compared with skeletal muscle, and the variation in cardiac tissue content of FABP is less than of myoglobin and similar to the variations found for HBDH or LDH.[194] H-FABP concentrations in human skeletal muscle are much lower than in heart. For myoglobin the situation is just the other way round, and, therefore, the myoglobin/H-FABP ratio markedly differs between heart and skeletal muscle (see Table 5.6). The ratio found in heart muscle is approximately 4-5, that found in skeletal muscle depends on the fiber-type composition of muscles and ranges from 20-70.[195] This different situation in heart and skeletal muscle tissue is also reflected by plasma concentrations of H-FABP and myoglobin after damage to striated muscles. As outlined below, the calculation of the myoglobin over H-FABP ratio from plasma concentrations after muscle damage allows to discriminate between heart and skeletal muscle with sufficient accuracy.

WHY COULD H-FABP BE MORE SENSITIVE THAN MYOGLOBIN?

H-FABP is not more specific than myoglobin for the diagnosis of myocardial injury, but for two reasons it could be more sensitive: (1) compared with myoglobin distribution between heart and skeletal muscle the tissue concentrations of H-FABP in heart are considerably higher and (2) H-FABP concentrations found in healthy people and patients without acute myocardial damage are much lower than for myoglobin (myoglobin usually <70 μg/L vs. H-FABP <4 μg/L).[192] This could improve the signal-to-noise ratio in patients with myocardial damage compared with myoglobin, in particular at the low range of concentrations.

CLINICAL RESULTS

Acute myocardial infarction

In a canine model of myocardial injury induced by coronary artery occlusion and reperfusion it could be demonstrated that H-FABP is an early indicator of myocardial injury.[196] In this myocardial injury model, plasma and urinary H-FABP levels showed a rapid increase after reperfusion. H-FABP was rapidly cleared by

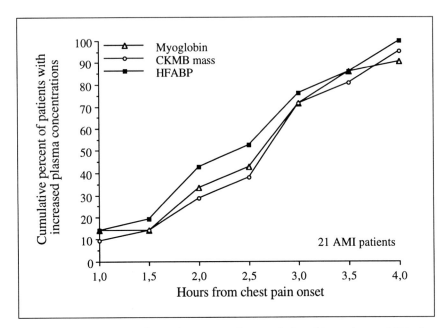

Fig. 5.37. First increases above the upper reference limits of heart fatty acid-binding protein, myoglobin, and CKMB mass concentrations after acute myocardial infarction (AMI). Study population: 21 AMI patients; delay from onset of chest pain to coronary care unit (CCU) admission: range 60-240 minutes; median 150 minutes. Nineteen patients showed unequivocal signs of myocardial ischemia (sensitivity: 0.90; 95%CI: 0.70-0.99) in their admission ECG recording and were treated with intravenous thrombolytic treatment; 12 Q wave, 7 aborted Q wave, and 2 non-Q wave AMI; 7 inferiorposterior and 14 anteriorlateral wall AMIs. Sensitivities at CCU admission: H-FABP 0.81 (95% confidence interval [CI]: 0.58-0.94), myoglobin 0.76 (95% CI: 0.53-0.89), CKMB mass 0.67 (95% CI: 0.43-0.85).

the kidneys. The plasma half-life time was approximately 30 minutes. Infarct size was closely correlated to calculated H-FABP release.

These experimental results could be confirmed in patients with AMI. H-FABP and myoglobin show a similar pattern of release into and clearance from plasma. FABP increases rapidly after AMI, usually between 2-4 hours (see Fig. 5.37), in parallel to myoglobin or CKMB mass. In our preliminary investigation there was no significant difference between the early sensitivities of H-FABP and myoglobin, although H-FABP tended to be somewhat more sensitive (see Fig. 5.37). H-FABP peak values occur about 5-10 hours after chest pain onset depending on reperfusion of the infarct-related coronary artery, usually in parallel to myoglobin (see Figs. 5.38, 5.39). Similar to myoglobin, the rate of increase is higher

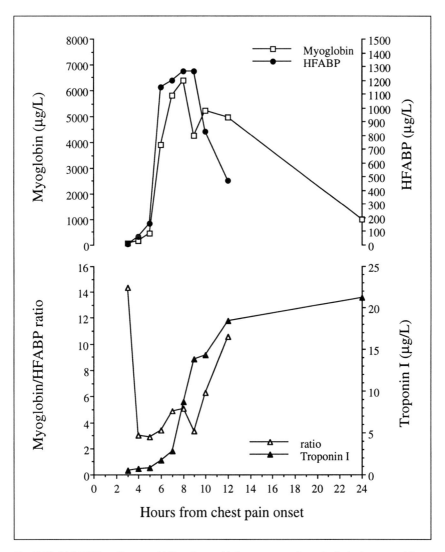

Fig. 5.38. H-FABP in a Q wave AMI patient with intravenous thrombolytic therapy without early reperfusion. This case illustrates a problem with the specificity of the myoglobin/ H-FABP ratio (calculated by simple division) in the early phase of AMI. In samples with moderately increased myoglobin and H-FABP the ratio may be much higher than five and is still within the range of values found in healthy subjects. In the first sample both myoglobin and H-FABP were slightly increased above the upper reference limit.

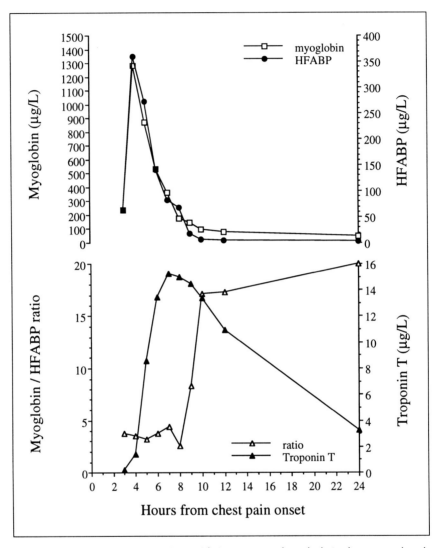

Fig. 5.39. H-FABP in a Q-wave AMI with intravenous thrombolytic therapy and early reperfusion of the infarct-related coronary artery. This case illustrates a problem with the specificity of the myoglobin/H-FABP ratio (calculated by simple division) in the later phase of AMI. In samples with still moderately increased myoglobin and H-FABP concentrations the ratio may be much higher than five and is back in the range of values found in healthy subjects. At 10 and 12 hours both myoglobin and H-FABP were still slightly increased. Thus, the ratio has a shorter diagnostic window than H-FABP or myoglobin alone.

and the peak values are found earlier in patients with early reperfusion (see Figs. 5.38, 5.39). Criteria for the discrimination of patients with and without early reperfusion remain to be established and evaluated in with acute coronary angiography controlled studies. Release of H-FABP was completed after 24-36 hours.[197] Infarct size estimated from the cumulative release of the proteins and expressed as gram equivalents of healthy myocardium per liter of plasma yielded comparable values for H-FABP, CKMB, and HBDH.[197] Urinary H-FABP is also elevated during the early phase of AMI.[198]

H-FABP in patients with unstable angina pectoris

Increases in H-FABP have been described similar to myoglobin in a subgroup of patients with unstable angina not fulfilling standard WHO AMI criteria.[198] No data on its prognostic significance in these patients are yet available.

H-FABP in patients undergoing coronary artery bypass grafting (CABG)

CABG is a complex clinical situation with myocardial and skeletal muscle injury (see chapter 2). Because skeletal muscle injury is mostly small and negligible as a source of false positive results, myoglobin was found to be a reliable and early predictor of the occurrence of perioperative myocardial infarction (PMI) (see myoglobin). Nonetheless the lack of cardiac specificity of myoglobin may raise doubts in the individual patient, which may be eliminated by the calculation of the myoglobin over H-FABP ratio. This ratio allows to define the major source of myoglobin and H-FABP release in CABG patients. Figure 5.40 demonstrates H-FABP, myoglobin and cardiac troponin I time courses in a representative patient undergoing CABG without PMI. This case nicely demonstrates the potential of the myoglobin/H-FABP ratio in CABG patients. During cardioplegic cardiac arrest (before aortic unclamping) the heart is bypassed by the heart lung machine and does not contribute to H-FABP release. The small skeletal muscle damage, caused by thoracotomy and preparation of the veins or internal mammary artery, causes a moderate increase in myoglobin from the skeletal muscle (high myoglobin/H-FABP ratio). However, after aortic unclamping when coronary artery blood flow is reestablished the ratio drops dramatically and indicates that the

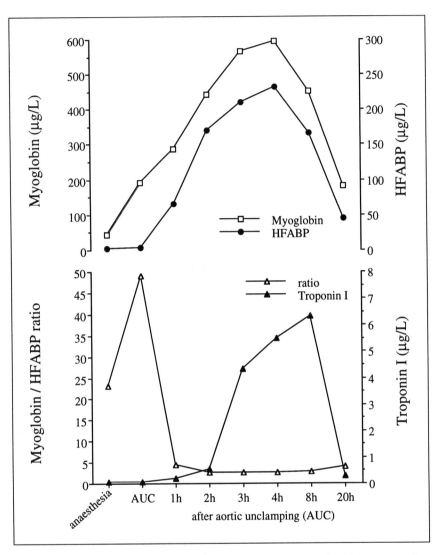

Fig. 5.40. H-FABP, myoglobin, and cardiac troponin I concentration time courses in a patient with coronary artery bypass grafting without perioperative myocardial infarction. This case nicely demonstrates the potential of the myoglobin/H-FABP ratio in CABG patients. During cardioplegic cardiac arrest (before aortic unclamping [AUC]) the heart is bypassed by the heart lung machine and does not contribute to H-FABP release. The small skeletal muscle damage caused by thoracotomy and preparation of the veins or internal mammary artery causes a moderate increase in myoglobin from the skeletal muscle (high myoglobin/H-FABP ratio). However after aortic unclamping, when coronary artery blood flow is reestablished, the ratio drops dramatically and indicates that the detectable myoglobin is released from the heart. This is confirmed by the cardiac troponin I time course. cTnI started to increase 1 hour after AUC.

detectable myoglobin and H-FABP is released from the heart. This is confirmed by the cardiac troponin I time course. cTnI started to increase 1 hour after aortic unclamping (see Fig. 5.40). In uncomplicated patients H-FABP peaks in parallel to myoglobin within 4 hours after AUC. Myoglobin and H-FABP serum concentration allow identification of PMI as early as 3 hours after aortic unclamping.

Diagnostic specificity of H-FABP: improved specificity by calculating the myoglobin over H-FABP ratio

From its tissue distribution it can be derived that H-FABP is not a more cardiac-specific marker than myoglobin. The two major sources of false positive results are skeletal muscle damage (see Fig. 5.41) and damage to the kidneys, because these two tissues contain considerable amounts of H-FABP. However, any condition with a decreased glomerular filtration rate causes increased H-FABP and myoglobin serum concentration, because these two proteins are primarily eliminated from blood by glomerular filtration, tubular reabsorption and subsequent catabolism in the tubular cells. If the reabsorptive capacity of the renal tubular system is saturated the excess of small proteins, such as H-FABP and myoglobin, will be excreted into the urine.

The diagnostic specificities of both myoglobin and H-FABP can be improved by the calculation of the myoglobin over H-FABP ratio (see Fig. 5.42), because the tissue ratios of myoglobin over H-FABP are reflected by the ratio of plasma concentrations after muscle damage (see above). The discrimination seems to be reliably possible at peak concentrations. The currently available data suggest a cut-off value between 8-10 for the discrimination of heart and skeletal muscle damage. The overlap is greater in the increasing and decreasing phase of protein release after muscle damage. For example, Figure 5.38 illustrates this problem with the specificity of the myoglobin/H-FABP ratio (calculated by simple division) in the early phase of AMI. In samples with moderately increased myoglobin and H-FABP the ratio may be much higher than five and is still within the range of values found in healthy subjects. Figure 5.39 illustrates the problem during the later phase of AMI. In samples with still moderately increased myoglobin and H-FABP concentrations the ratio may be much higher than five

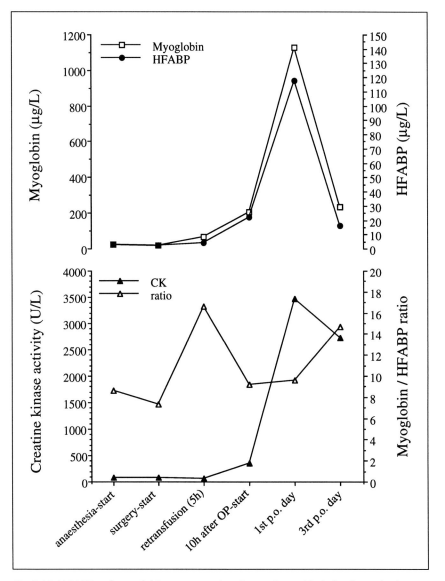

Fig. 5.41. H-FABP and myoglobin concentrations in a patient with skeletal muscle damage after orthopedic surgery (posterioranterior fusion). Cardiac troponin I was not detectable in any sample taken.

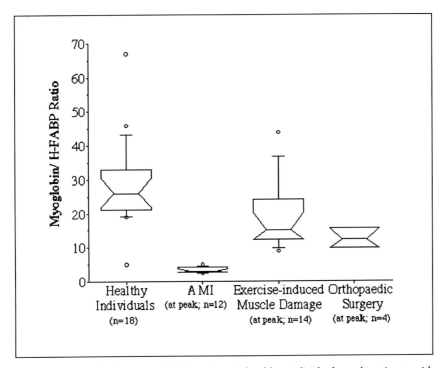

Fig. 5.42. Myoglobin over H-FABP ratios in healthy individuals and patients with myocardial or skeletal muscle damage. The discrimination seems to be reliably possible at peak concentrations. The currently available data suggest a cut-off value of 8-10 for the discrimination of heart and skeletal muscle damage. The overlap is greater in the increasing and decreasing phase of protein release after muscle damage.

and is back in the range of values found in healthy subjects. Thus, the ratio has a shorter diagnostic window than H-FABP or myoglobin alone. The discrimination between heart and skeletal muscle damage seems to be far more problematic in samples with only slightly to moderately increased myoglobin and H-FABP concentrations, and therefore the calculation of this ratio is also not useful in patients with unstable angina.

CLINICAL USE OF H-FABP—SUMMARY

H-FABP, like myoglobin, is a sensitive marker especially for the early assessment or exclusion of AMI. Recent preliminary data from the European multicenter trial on the use of H-FABP in the early evaluation of patients with acute coronary syndromes (J. Glatz et al, unpublished data) suggest that H-FABP is more sensitive for the detection of AMI than myoglobin in patients (n = 86) admitted within 6 hours from chest pain onset (sensitivities: myoglobin 0.53, H-FABP 0.77). However, we could not confirm this large difference in our own AMI population investigated (see Fig. 5.37). It remains to be seen whether this difference in the early sensitivities of myoglobin and H-FABP is large enough to gain significance for clinical practice. Comparative studies between GPBB and H-FABP are required as well. But H-FABP is undoubtedly at least as sensitive as myoglobin. Similar to myoglobin, its rapid elimination from plasma under normal conditions makes H-FABP a suitable marker for the detection of recurrent infarctions.

The interference of possible skeletal muscle damage can be assessed and partly eliminated from calculating the ratio of plasma concentrations of myoglobin and FABP. This ratio, however, appears to be less reliable for the discrimination of heart and skeletal muscle injury at slightly to moderately increased serum concentrations of both markers. There is no doubt that this ratio cannot provide absolute cardiac specificity, similar to the CKMB/CK ratio. In patients with suspected myocardial injury with overt or possible skeletal muscle damage clearly cardiac-specific markers, such as cardiac troponin I and troponin T, are to be preferred to assess myocardial involvement. Fortunately, in the nontraumatic chest pain patient skeletal muscle damage is a rare complication, and the real problem is missing the diagnosis AMI because of lack of early sensitivities of markers.

In summary, according to current knowledge and data H-FABP is an equivalent marker to myoglobin for the diagnosis of myocardial injury. It can be measured instead or also in combination with myoglobin. However, H-FABP assays which are suitable for use in the emergency laboratory or bedside tests are not yet available.

MYOGLOBIN OVER CARBONIC ANHYDRASE ISOENZYME III RATIO

Measurement of carbonic anhydrase isoenzyme III (CA III) and calculation of the myoglobin over CA III ratio is another way proposed for increasing the specificity of myoglobin measurements for the diagnosis of myocardial injury. CA III is a soluble protein (MW: 29 kDa) and has been shown to exist, in contrast to myoglobin, in high amounts only in skeletal muscle and not in the myocardium.[199,200]

BIOCHEMISTRY

The carbonic anhydrases (CA) efficiently catalyze the hydration of CO_2 to bicarbonate and a proton. There are seven CA isoenzymes (I-VII) which are encoded by a gene family (reviewed in ref. 200). All seven isoenzymes have been cloned, sequenced and mapped. The seven isoenzymes differ in kinetics, subcellular localization, and in tissue-specific distribution. CAs participate in a variety of physiological processes that involve pH regulation, CO_2 and bicarbonate transport, ion transport, and water and electrolyte balance. Metabolic roles include important steps in ureagenesis, gluconeogenesis, and lipogenesis. The diversity among different CA isoenzymes is large enough to produce CA III specific antibodies.[201]

The major site of CA III expression is skeletal muscle, where it can represent 8% of the soluble protein of slow-twitch (type I fiber) red skeletal muscle. It is expressed in other fiber-types in much lower amounts. CA III is also expressed at low levels in salivary glands, smooth muscle cells in uterus, erythrocytes, prostate, lung, kidney, colon, and testis.[200] Most importantly CA III is not expressed in human myocardium.[199,200]

RATIONALE OF MEASURING CA III IN PATIENTS WITH SUSPECTED MYOCARDIAL INJURY

The simultaneous measurement of serum myoglobin and CA III can be used to differentiate between myocardial and skeletal muscle damage. The ratio of serum myoglobin over CA III originating from skeletal muscle stays fairly constant after skeletal muscle damage, but increases after injury to the myocardium,[202] because unlike myoglobin it is not found in cardiac muscle. This can be used as an aid to identify the source of myoglobin when it is elevated in the serum.

DIAGNOSTIC SPECIFICITY OF MYOGLOBIN OVER CA III RATIO

After skeletal muscle damage CA III correlates closely with myoglobin release. It increases, peaks and disappears in parallel to myoglobin after skeletal muscle damage. For example, CA III is increased in patients with neuromuscular diseases and in healthy subjects after physical exercise.[202] Peak values of CA III and myoglobin occur in parallel and correlate closely.[202] The diagnostic specificity for skeletal muscle damage is high. The myoglobin/CA III ratio remains constant after skeletal muscle damage because both proteins are released from the damaged muscle. In contrast to myoglobin, CA III does not increase in AMI patients and the ratio increases.

In a study investigating 251 consecutive nontraumatic chest pain patients[203] Brogan et al found that the myoglobin/CA III ratio was significantly more sensitive for AMI detection than CKMB mass in patients admitted within 3 hours of symptom onset and that the calculation of the ratio could improve the specificity of myoglobin by reducing the number of false positive myoglobin results. Specificities of myoglobin/CA III ratio and CKMB mass were comparable. However, in another study[204] investigating 267 chest pain patients without trauma the diagnostic accuracy of myoglobin, myoglobin/CA III ratio and CKMB or CKMB/CK ratio did not differ significantly. The calculation of the myoglobin/CA III ratio could not significantly increase the specificity of myoglobin measurements, which illustrates that in the population of the nontraumatic chest pain patients skeletal muscle damage is rare enough not to significantly affect the diagnostic accuracy of myoglobin.

CLINICAL USEFULNESS OF MEASURING CA III—SUMMARY

CA III assays are not yet commercially available. The currently available data suggest that by the means of myoglobin over CA III ratio of serum concentrations it may be possible to discriminate between heart and skeletal muscle damage. However, this hypothesis was tested only in selected patient populations so far. The general usefulness of CA III measurement needs to be confirmed in larger trials, including unselected patients with, for example, renal failure, cocaine use, trauma and rhabdomyolysis.[203] In renal failure CA III is expected to be increased similar to myoglobin or heart fatty acid binding protein. Similar to the CKMB/CK and myoglobin/H-FABP ratios, the myoglobin/CA III ratio will hardly provide absolute cardiac specificity. In the patient with real or possible concomitant skeletal muscle damage cardiac troponin I and troponin T are the markers of choice for determining myocardial damage.

On the other hand, in the nontraumatic chest pain patients concomitant skeletal muscle damage is rare, and there is no need for CA III measurement when skeletal muscle damage can be clinically excluded. This is nicely illustrated by the fact that myoglobin/CA III ratio was not significantly more specific than myoglobin in the study of Vuori et al.[204]

In summary, myoglobin/CA III ratio will not become important for the diagnosis of myocardial injury in presence of skeletal muscle damage. CA III may gain significance as a marker of skeletal muscle injury in athletes or patients with muscular diseases.

OTHER MARKERS WITH LIMITED AVAILABLE CLINICAL DATA

Besides the already discussed parameters a number of additional markers have been proposed as diagnostic markers for myocardial injury. For all parameters dealt with in this chapter, assays are not commercially available. The available clinical data are very limited and a judgment of their diagnostic accuracy is currently not possible. The presentation will, therefore, be focused on their biochemical basis and on first clinical results, if they are available.

PHOSPHOGLYCERIC ACID MUTASE ISOENZYME MB

Human phosphoglyceric acid mutase (PGAM) is a dimer comprising MM, BB, and MB isoenzymes. It is a glycolytic enzyme and catalyzes the interconversion between 2- and 3-phosphoglycerate in the presence of the cofactor 2,3-biphosphoglycerate.[205] The dimer is formed from the muscle-specific (M) and nonmuscle-specific (B) subunits. Both subunits have a MW of approximately 30 kDa and are encoded by different genes. Specific antibodies against the M and B subunit have been developed,[205] and currently an immunoassay for measurement of the MB isoenzyme of PGAM is being developed by a Japanese group. The MB isoenzyme of PGAM has been proposed as a marker for myocardial damage.[205]

The BB isoenzyme (B-type) is found in adult brain, liver, kidney, and erythrocytes. The MM isoenzyme (M-type) is expressed in adult skeletal and cardiac muscles. In the heart also a MB heterodimer is formed, the MB isoenzyme (MB-type). In fetal and neonatal skeletal muscles, the B-type and MB-type are formed in addition to the M-type.[206] The M-type also exists in certain neoplasmas of the brain where the level of expression appears to be correlated with the degree of malignancy of the tumor.[205]

The PGAM enzyme activity found in plasma of normal subjects was exclusively due to the B-type, whereas the activity in the plasma of patients with Duchenne muscular dystrophy was due to a mixture of the M and B-type.[207]

From its tissue distribution and its expression pattern in diseases it can be derived that PGAM isoenzyme MB is not a heart-specific marker. No comment on its diagnostic sensitivity for myocardial infarction and injury is currently possible, because there are no published experimental or clinical data.

ENOLASE ISOENZYME $\alpha\beta$

Enolase is another glycolytic enzyme abundantly present in all tissues. It catalyzes the interconversion of 2-phosphoglycerate and phosphoenolpyruvate. The enzyme exists as a dimeric structure composed of three distinct subunits, with a MW of approximately 90 kDa. Each subunit is encoded by different genes.[208] Five isoenzymes of enolase have been described ($\alpha\alpha$, $\alpha\beta$, $\beta\beta$, $\alpha\gamma$ and $\gamma\gamma$) with the $\alpha\beta$-enolase as the predominant form in the myocardium and $\beta\beta$-enolase in skeletal muscle.[208] $\alpha\gamma$ and $\gamma\gamma$ isoenzymes are found in neuronal tissues. Increases in total enolase activity and β-enolase have been described in AMI patients and patients undergoing cardiac surgery.[209-211] After AMI enolase increases, peaks and decreases in parallel to CKMB.[209,210] Like CK, enolase undergoes postsynthetic modifications in plasma.[212]

Measurement of β-enolase will not enable differentiation of skeletal muscle and cardiac muscle damage. A specific assay for $\alpha\beta$-enolase might be possibly more useful. However, even this strategy may not result in a heart-specific marker if diseases that affect either the myocardium or skeletal muscle alter the distribution of enolase isoenzymes. At present it appears that the sensitivities and specificities of CKMB and $\alpha\beta$-enolase are comparable. Therefore, this marker will probably not gain significance for the laboratory diagnosis of myocardial injury.

S100a$_0$ PROTEIN

Protein S100, an acidic and calcium-binding protein, belongs to a family of proteins, which also includes calmodulin, troponin C, parvalbumin, and myosin light chain. S100 is a dimeric protein which consists of two different subunits (α and β). There are three isoforms $\alpha\alpha$ (S100a$_0$), $\alpha\beta$ (S100a) and $\beta\beta$ (S100b). Protein S100 is present in cardiac as well as in skeletal muscle and most abundantly in glial cells.[213] S100a$_0$ protein (MW 21 kDa) is present in high concentrations in myocardium and skeletal muscle.[213,214]

Increased S100a$_0$ concentrations in serum have been described in AMI patients, after open heart surgery, and patients with muscular dystrophy.[215,216] After AMI it rises within a few hours, peaks at about 8 hours and stays, in contrast to myoglobin and CKMB, elevated for several days.[215] S100a$_0$ is mostly eliminated from blood by the kidneys. It is excreted in the urine and its biological half-life is shorter than that of serum CKMB.[216] Therefore its prolonged increase is explained by continuing release from cardiomyocytes. S100a$_0$ is known to be associated with various structural elements in the muscle fiber (e.g., the intercalated disc).[215] The characteristic localization of S100a$_0$ in the myocardium obviously results in its prompt and continuing release from infarcted myocardium. In patients with unstable angina increased S100a$_0$ ($\alpha\alpha$) serum concentrations were not found.[215]

In summary, S100a$_0$ is not a heart-specific marker. It increases rapidly after AMI as does myoglobin. In contrast to myoglobin it stays elevated for several days. However, it is not likely that S100a$_0$ will play a major role in the laboratory diagnosis of myocardial injury, because more suitable markers are already available.

REFERENCES

1. Zweig MH, van Steirteghem AC, Schechter AN. Radioimmunoassays of creatine kinase isoenzymes in human serum: isoenzyme BB. Clin Chem 1978; 24:422-8.
2. Neumeier D, Hofstetter R, Gluck B. Radioimmunoassays for subunit B in isoenzymes CK-MB and CK-BB of creatine phosphokinase. Clin Chim Acta 1977; 79:107-13.
3. Depuey EG, Aessopos A, Monroe LR et al. Clinical utility of a two-site immunoradiometric assay for creatine kinase MB in the detection of perioperative myocardial infarction. J Nucl Med 1983; 24:703-9.
4. Bhayana V, Henderson AR. Biochemical markers of myocardial damage. Clin Biochem 1995; 28:1-29.
5. Chan KM, Ladenson JH, Pierce GF, Jaffe AS. Increased creatine kinase MB in the absence of acute myocardial infarction. Clin Chem 1986; 32:2044-51.
6. Vaidya H, Apple F, Boches F et al. Standardization of creatine kinase-MB (CKMB) mass immunoassays (abstract). Clin Biochem

1993; 14:337.

7. Al-Sheik W, Heal AV, Pefkaros KC et al. Evaluation of an immunoradiometric assay specific for the CK-MB isoenzyme for detection of acute myocardial infarction. Am J Cardiol 1984; 54:269-73.

8. Eisenberg PR, Shaw D, Schaab C, Jaffe AS. Concordance of creatine kinase-MB activity and mass. Clin Chem 1989; 35:440-3.

9. Gibler WB, Lewis LM, Erb RE et al. Early detection of acute myocardial infarction in patients presenting with chest pain and nondiagnostic ECGs: serial CKMB sampling in the emergency department. Ann Emerg Med 1990:19:1359-66.

10. Mair J, Artner-Dworzak A, Dienstl A et al. Early detection of acute myocardial infarction by measurement of mass concentration of creatine kinase-MB. Am J Cardiol 1991; 68:1545-50.

11. Collinson PO, Rosalki SB, Kuwana T et al. Early diagnosis of acute myocardial infarction by CK-MB mass measurements. Ann Clin Biochem 1992; 29:43-7.

12. Mair J, Morandell D, Genser N et al. Equivalent early sensitivities of myoglobin, creatine kinase MB mass, creatine kinase isoform ratios, and cardiac troponins I and T for acute myocardial infarction. Clin Chem 1995; 41:1266-72.

13. Gibler WB, Runyon JP, Levy RC et al. A rapid diagnostic and treatment center for patients with chest pain in the emergency department. Ann Emerg Med 1995; 25:1-8.

14. Mair J, Smidt J, Lechleitner P, Dienstl F, Puschendorf B. Rapid accurate diagnosis of acute myocardial infarction in non-traumatic chest pain within 1 hour after admission. Coronary Artery Dis 1995; 6:539-45.

15. Marin MM, Teichman SL. Use of rapid serial sampling of creatine kinase MB for very early detection of myocardial infarction in patients with acute chest pain. Am Heart J 1992; 123:354-61.

16. Apple FS. Acute myocardial infarction and coronary reperfusion. Serum cardiac markers for the 1990s. Am J Clin Pathol 1992; 97:217-26.

17. Zabel M, Hohnloser SH, Köster W et al. Analysis of creatine kinase, CK-MB, myoglobin, and troponin T time-activity curves for early assessment of coronary artery reperfusion after intravenous thrombolysis. Circulation 1993; 87:1542-50.

18. Garabedian HD, Gold HK, Yasuda T et al. Detection of coronary artery reperfusion with creatine kinase-MB determination during thrombolytic therapy: correlation with acute angiography. J Am Coll Cardiol 1988; 11:729-34.

19. Laperche T, Steg PG, Dehoux M et al. A study of biochemical markers of reperfusion early after thrombolysis for acute myocardial infarction. Circulation 1995; 92:2079-86.

20. Ravkilde J, Nissen H, Horder M, Thygesen K. Independent prog-

nostic value of serum creatine kinase isoenzyme mass, cardiac troponin T and myosin light chain levels in suspected acute myocardial infarction. J Am Coll Cardiol 1995; 25:574-81.

21. Ravkilde J, Bo Hansen A, Jorgenson PL, Thygesen K. Risk stratification in suspected acute myocardial infarction based on a sensitive immunoassay for serum creatine kinase isoenzyme MB. Cardiology 1992; 80:143-51.

22. Chapelle JP, El Allaf D, El Allaf M et al. Serum creatine kinase isoenzyme MB concentration after endomyocardial biopsy. Clin Chim Acta 157;1986:55-64.

23. Ravkilde J, Nissen H, Mickley H et al. Cardiac troponin T and CKMB mass release after visually successful percutaneous transluminal coronary angioplasty in stable angina pectoris. Am Heart J 1994; 127:13-20.

24. Talasz H, Genser N, Mair J et al. Side branch occlusion during percutaneous transluminal coronary angioplasty. Lancet 1992; 339:1380-2.

25. Lee Th, Goldmann L. Serum enzyme assays in the diagnosis of acute myocardial infarction. Ann Intern Med 1986; 105:221-33.

26. Gulbis B, Unger P, Lenaers A et al. Mass concentration of creatine kinase MB isoenzyme and lactate dehydrogenase isoenzyme 1 in diagnosis of perioperative myocardial infarction after coronary bypass surgery. Clin Chem 1990; 36:1784-8.

27. Chapelle JP, El Allaf M, Larbuisson R et al. The value of serum CK-MB and myoglobin for assessing perioperative myocardial infarction after cardiac surgery. Scand J Clin Lab Invest 1986; 46:519-26.

28. Mair P, Mair J, Seibt I et al. Creatine kinase isoenzyme MB mass concentrations in patients undergoing aortocoronary bypass surgery. Clin Chim Acta 1994; 224:203-7.

29. Puleo PR, Meyer D, Wathen C et al. Use of a rapid assay of subforms of creatine kinase MB to diagnose or rule out acute myocardial infarction. New Engl J Med 1994; 331:561-6.

30. Wevers RA, Wolters RJ, Soons JBJ. Isoelectric focusing and hybridisation experiments on creatine kinase. Clin Chim Acta 1977; 78:271-6.

31. Heinbokel N, Strivastava LM, Goedde HW. Agarose gel isoelectric focusing of creatine kinase isoenzymes from different human tissue extracts. Clin Chim Acta 1982; 122:103-7.

32. Edwards RJ, Watts DC. Human creatine kinase conversion factor identified as a carboxypeptidase. Biochem J 1984; 221:465-70.

33. Perryman MB, Knell JD, Roberts R. Carboxypeptidase-catalyzed hydrolysis of C-terminal lysine: mechanism for in vivo production of multiple forms of creatine kinase in plasma. Clin Chem 1984; 30:662-4.

34. Billadello JJ, Fontanet HL, Strauss AW et al. Characterization of

MB creatine kinase isoform conversion in vitro and in vivo in dogs. J Clin Invest 1989; 83:1637-43.

35. Kanemitsu F, Okigaki T. Characterization of human creatine kinase BB and MB isoforms by means of isoelectric focusing. Clin Chim Acta 1994; 231:1-9.

36. Puleo PR, Guadagno PA, Roberts R et al. Sensitive, rapid assay of subforms of creatine kinase MB in plasma. Clin Chem 1989; 35:1452-55.

37. Bhayana V, Cohoe S, Leung FY et al. Diagnostic evaluation of creatine kinase-2 mass and creatine kinase-3 and -2 isoform ratios in early diagnosis of acute myocardial infarction. Clin Chem 1993; 39:488-95.

38. Hossein-Nia M, Kallis P, Brown PA et al. Creatine kinase MB isoforms: sensitive markers of ischemic myocardial damage. Clin Chem 1994; 40:1265-71.

39. Davies D, Reynolds T, Penney MD. Creatine kinase isoforms: investigation of inhibitors of in vitro degradation and establishment of a reference range. Ann Clin Biochem 1992; 29:202-5.

40. Kanemitsu F, Okigaki T. A combination assay of MB and MM isoforms of serum creatine kinase in acute myocardial infarction. Clin Chim Acta 1994; 229:161-9.

41. Prager NA, Suzuki T, Jaffe AS et al. Nature and time course of generation of isoforms of creatine kinase MB fraction in vivo. J Am Coll Cardiol 1992; 20:414-9.

42. Abendschein DR, Fontanet HL, Nohara R. Optimized preservation of creatine kinase MM isoenzyme in plasma specimens and their rapid quantification by semi-automated chromatofocusing. Clin Chem 1990; 36:723-7.

43. Wu AHB. Creatine kinase isoforms in ischemic heart disease. Clin Chem 1989; 35:7-13.

44. Panteghini M, Bonora R, Pagani F. An immunoinhibition assay for determination of creatine kinase isoforms in serum. Eur J Clin Chem Clin Biochem 1994; 32:383-9.

45. Christenson RH, Ohman EM, Topol EJ et al. Creatine kinase MM and MB isoforms in patients receiving thrombolytic therapy and acute angiography. Clin Chem 1995; 41:844-52.

46. George S, Ishikawa Y, Perryman MB et al. Purification and characterization of naturally occurring and in vitro induced forms of creatine kinase. J Biol Chem 1984; 259:2667-74.

47. Erdös EG, Skidgel RA. More on subforms of creatine kinase MB (letter). New Engl J Med 1995; 333:390.

48. Wittenberg JB. Myoglobin-facilitated oxygen diffusion: role of myoglobin in oxygen entry into muscle. Physiol Rev 1970; 50:559-636.

49. Braunlin EA, Wahler GM, Swayze CR et al. Myoglobin facilitated oxygen diffusion maintains mechanical function of mammalian car-

diac muscle. Cardiovasc Res 1986; 20:627-36.

50. Wu JT, Pieper RK, Wu LH, Peters JL. Isolation and characterization of myoglobin and its two major isoforms from sheep heart. Clin Chem 1989; 35:778-82.

51. Stone MJ, Willerson JT, Gomez-Sanchez CE et al. Radioimmunoassay of myoglobin in human serum. Results in patients with acute myocardial infarction. J Clin Invest 1975; 56:1334-9.

52. Delanghe J, Chapelle JP, Vanderschueren S. Quantitative nephelometric assay for determining myoglobin evaluated. Clin Chem 1990; 36:1675-8.

53. Mair J, Artner-Dworzak E, Lechleitner P et al. Early diagnosis of acute myocardial infarction by a newly developed rapid immunoturbidimetric assay for myoglobin. Br Heart J 1992; 68:462-8.

54. de Winter RJ, Koster RW, Sturk A, Sanders GT. Value of myoglobin, troponin T, and CKMB mass in ruling out an acute myocardial infarction in the emergency room. Circulation 1995; 92:3401-7.

55. Klocke FJ, Copley DP, Krawczyk JA et al. Rapid renal clearance of immunoreactive canine plasma myoglobin. Circulation 1982; 65:1522-8.

56. Yamashita T, Abe S, Arima S et al. Myocardial infarct size can be estimated from serial plasma myoglobin measurements within 4 hours of reperfusion. Circulation 1993; 87:1840-9.

57. Honda Y, Katayama T. Detection of myocardial infarction extension or reattack by serum myoglobin radioimmunoassay. Int J Cardiol 1984; 6:325-35.

58. Ohman EM, Casey C, Bengtson JR et al. Early detection of acute myocardial infarction: additional diagnostic information from serum concentrations of myoglobin in patients without ST elevation. Br Heart J 1990; 63:335-8.

59. Miyata M, Abe S, Arima S et al. Rapid diagnosis of coronary reperfusion by measurement of myoglobin level every 15 min in acute myocardial infarction. J Am Coll Cardiol 1994; 23:1009-15.

60. Abe S, Arima S, Nomoto K et al. Early detection of coronary reperfusion by rapid assessment of plasma myoglobin. Int J Cardiol 1993; 38:33-40.

61. The TIMI study group. The thrombolysis in myocardial infarction (TIMI) trial. New Engl J Med 1985; 311:932-6.

62. Mair P, Mair J, Seibt I et al. Early and rapid diagnosis of perioperative myocardial infarction in aortocoronary bypass surgery by immunoturbidimetric myoglobin measurements. Chest 1993; 103:1508-11.

63. Seguin Saussine M, Ferriere M et al. Comparison of myoglobin and creatine kinase MB levels in the evaluation of myocardial injury after cardiac operations. J Thorac Cardiovasc Surg 1988; 95:294-7.

64. Kinoshita K, Tsuruhara Y, Tokunaga K. Delayed time to peak serum myoglobin level as an indicator of cardiac dysfunction following open heart surgery. Chest 1991; 99:1398-402.

65. Hoberg E, Katus HA, Diederich KW, Kübler W. Myoglobin, creatine kinase-B isoenzyme, and myosin light chain release in patients with unstable angina pectoris. Eur Heart J 1987; 8:989-94.

66. Isakov A, Shapira I, Burke M, Almog C. Serum myoglobin levels in patients with ischemic myocardial insult. Arch Intern Med 1988; 148:1762-5.

67. Roxin LE, Cullhed I, Groth T et al. The value of serum myoglobin determinations in the early diagnosis of acute myocardial infarction. Acta Med Scand 1984; 215:417-21.

68. Hart PM, Feinfeld DA, Briscoe AM et al. The effect of renal failure and hemodialysis on serum and urine myoglobin. Clin Nephrology 1982; 18:141-3.

69. Sabria M, Ruibal A, Rey C et al. Influence of exercise on serum myoglobin levels measured by radioimmunoassay. Eur J Nucl Med 1983; 8:159-61.

70. Balnave CD, Thompson MW. Effect of training on eccentric exercise-induced muscle damage. J Appl Physiol 1993; 75:1545-51.

71. Wu AHB, Laios I, Green S et al. Immunoassays for serum and urine myoglobin: myoglobin clearance assessed as a risk factor for acute renal failure. Clin Chem 1994; 40:796-802.

72. Farah CS, Reinach FC. The troponin complex and regulation of muscle contraction. FASEB J 1995; 9:755-67.

73. Raggi A, Grand RJA, Moir AJG, Perry SV. Structure-function relationships in cardiac troponin T. Biochim Biophys Acta 1989; 997:135-43.

74. Pharmacek MS, Leiden JM. Structure, function and regulation of troponin C. Circulation 1991; 84:991-1003.

75. Harrington WF, Rodgers ME. Myosin. Ann Rev Biochem 53;1984:35-73.

76. Warrick HM, Spudich JA. Myosin structure and function in cell motility. Ann Rev Cell Biol 3;1987:379-421.

77. Cooke R. The actomyosin engine. FASEB J 1995; 9:636-42.

78. Yamauchi-Takihara K, Sole MJ et al. Characterization of human cardiac myosin heavy chain genes. Proc Natl Acad Sci USA 1989; 86:3504-8.

79. Barton PJR, Cohen A, Robert B et al. The myosin alkali light chains of mouse ventricular and slow skeletal muscle are indistinguishable and are encoded by the same gene. J Biol Chem 1984; 260:8578-84.

80. Collins JH, Theibert JL, Libera LD. Amino acid sequence of rabbit ventricular myosin light chain-2: identity with slow skeletal muscle isoform. Biosci Rep 1986; 6:655-71.

81. Schwartz K, Boheler KR, de la Bastie D et al. Switches in cardiac muscle gene expression as a result of pressure and volume over-

load. Am J Physiol 1992; 262:R364-9.

82. Cummins P. The homology of the alpha chains of cardiac and skeletal rabbit tropomyosin. J Mol Cell Cardiol 1979; 11:109-14.

83. Pearlstone J, Carpenter M, Smillie L. Amino acid sequences of rabbit cardiac troponin T. J Biol Chem 1986; 261:16795-810.

84. Wilkinson JM, Grand RJA. Comparison of amino acid sequence of troponin I from different striated muscles. Nature 1978; 271:31-5.

85. Boheler KR, Carrier L, de la Bastie D et al. Skeletal actin mRNA increases in the human heart during ontogenic development and is the major isoform of control and failing adult hearts. J Clin Invest 1991; 88:323-30.

86. Aranega AE, Reine A, Velez C et al. Circulating alpha-actin in angina pectoris. J Mol Cell Cardiol 1993; 25:15-22.

87. Cummins P, McGurk B, and Littler WA. Radioimmunoassay of human cardiac tropomyosin in acute myocardial infarction. Clin Science 1981; 60:251-9.

88. Anderson PAW, Malouf NN, Oakeley AE et al. Troponin T isoform expression in humans. A comparison among normal and failing adult heart, fetal heart, and adult and fetal skeletal muscle. Circ Res 1991; 69:1226-33.

89. Katus HA, Looser S, Hallermayer K et al. Development and in vitro characterization of a new immunoassay of cardiac troponin T. Clin Chem 1992; 38:386-93.

90. Katus HA, Remppis A, Scheffold T et al. Intracellular compartmentation of cardiac troponin T and its release kinetics in patients with reperfused and nonreperfused myocardial infarction. Am J Cardiol 1991; 67:1360-7.

91. Adams III JE, Bodor GS, Davila-Roman VG et al. Cardiac troponin I. A marker with high specificity for cardiac injury. Circulation 1993; 88:101-6.

92. Saggin L, Gorza L, Ausoni S, Schiaffino S. Cardiac troponin T in developing, regenerating and denerved rat skeletal muscle. Development 1990; 110:547-54.

93. Bodor G, Porterfield D, Voss E et al. Cardiac troponin T composition in regenerating human skeletal muscle tissue (abstract). Clin Chem 1995; 41:148.

94. Katus HA, Müller-Bardorff M, Hallermayer K et al. The second generation of the cardiac troponin T ELISA: improved specificity (abstract). Clin Chem 1995; 41:S79.

95. Mair J, Artner-Dworzak E, Lechleitner P et al. Cardiac troponin T in diagnosis of acute myocardial infarction. Clin Chem 1991; 37:845-52.

96. Katus HA, Remppis A, Neumann FJ et al. Diagnostic efficiency of troponin T measurements in acute myocardial infarction. Circulation 1991; 83:902-12.

97. Gerhardt W, Katus H, Ravkilde J et al. S-troponin T in suspected ischemic myocardial injury compared with mass and catalytic concentrations of S-creatine kinase isoenzyme MB. Clin Chem 1991; 37:1405-11.

98. Westfall MV, Solaro RJ. Alterations in myofibrillar function and protein profiles after complete global ischemia in rat hearts. Circulation Res 1990; 70:302-13.

99. Di Lisa F, de Tullio R, Salamino F et al. Specific degradation of troponin T and I by μ-calpain and its modulation by substrate phosphorylation. Biochem J 1995; 308:57-61.

100. Müller-Bardorff M, Freitag H, Scheffold T, Remppis A, Kübler W, Katus HA. Development and characterization of a rapid assay for bedside determinations of cardiac troponin T. Circulation 1995; 92:2869-75.

101. Abe S, Arima S, Yamashita T et al. Early assessment of reperfusion therapy using cardiac troponin T. J Am Coll Cardiol 1994; 23:1382-9.

102. Remppis A, Scheffold T, Karrer O et al. Assessment of reperfusion of the infarct zone after acute myocardial infarction by serial cardiac troponin T measurements in serum. Br Heart J 1994; 71:242-8.

103. Wagner I, Mair J, Fridrich L et al. Cardiac troponin T release in acute myocardial infarction is associated with scintigraphic estimates of myocardial scar. Coronary Artery Dis 1993; 4:537-44.

104. Omura T, Teragaki M, Tani T et al. Estimation of infarct size using serum troponin T concentration in patients with acute myocardial infarction. Jpn Circ J 1993; 57:1062-70.

105. Mair J, Genser N, Morandell D et al. Cardiac troponin I in the diagnosis of myocardial injury and infarction. Clin Chim Acta 1996; 245:19-38.

106. Mair J, Wieser C, Seibt I et al. Troponin T to diagnose myocardial infarction in bypass surgery. Lancet 1991; 337:434-5.

107. Katus HA, Schoeppenthau M, Tanzeem A et al. Non-invasive assessment of perioperative myocardial cell damage by circulating cardiac troponin T. Br Heart J 1991; 65:259-64.

108. Mair P, Mair J, Seibt I et al. Cardiac troponin T: a new marker of myocardial tissue damage in bypass surgery. J Cardiothor Vasc Anesth 1993; 7:674-8.

109. Eikvar L, Pillgram-Larsen J, Skjaeggestad O et al. Serum cardiospecific troponin T after open heart surgery in patients with and without perioperative myocardial infarction. Scand J Clin Lab Invest 1994; 54:329-35.

110. Hake U, Schmid FX, Iversen S et al. Troponin T—a reliable marker of perioperative myocardial infarction. Eur J Cardio-thorac Surg 1993; 7:628-33.

111. Hamm CW, Ravkilde J, Gerhardt W et al. The prognostic value of serum troponin T in unstable angina. New Engl J Med 1992;

327:146-50.

112. Ohman EM, Armstrong P, Califf RM et al. Risk stratification in acute ischaemic syndromes using serum troponin T (abstract). J Am Coll Cardiol 1995; 25:148A.

113. Lindahl B, Toss H, Venge P, Wallentin L. Troponin T is an independent prognostic marker for subsequent cardiac events in patients with unstable coronary artery disease (abstract). Circulation 1995; 92(suppl 1):3182.

114. Talasz H, Genser N, Mair J et al. Side-branch occlusion during percutaneous transluminal coronary angioplasty. Lancet 1992; 339:1380-2.

115. Ravkilde J, Nissen H, Mickley H et al. Cardiac troponin T and CKMB mass release after visually successful percutaneous transluminal coronary angioplasty in stable angina pectoris. Am Heart J 1994; 127:13-20.

116. Bachmaier K, Mair J, Offner F et al. Serum cardiac troponin T and creatine kinase-MB elevations in murine autoimmune myocarditis. Circulation 1995; 92:1927-32.

117. Mair J, Dienstl F, Puschendorf B. Cardiac troponin T in the diagnosis of myocardial injury. Crit Rev Clin Lab Sci 1992; 29:31-57.

118. Walpoth BH, Tschopp A, Peheim E et al. Assessment of troponin T for detection of cardiac rejection in a rat model. Transplant Proc 1995; 27:2084-7.

119. Zimmermann R, Baki S, Dengler TJ et al. Troponin T release after heart transplantation. Br Heart J 1993; 69:395-8.

120. Riou B, Dreux S, Roche S et al. Circulating cardiac troponin T in potential heart transplant donors. Circulation 1995; 92:409-14.

121. Mair P, Mair J, Koller J et al. Cardiac troponin T release in multiply injured patients. Injury 1995; 26:439-43.

122. Kobayashi S, Tanaka M, Tamura N et al. Serum cardiac troponin T in polymyositis/dermatomyositis (letter). Lancet 1992; 340:726.

123. Thome-Kromer B, Michel G. Human cardiac troponin I—detectability after myocardial infarction and severe skeletal muscle damage (abstract). Clin Chem 1993; 39:1248

124. Hafner G, Thome-Kromer B, Schaube J et al. Cardiac troponins in serum in chronic renal failure. Clin Chem 1994; 40:1790-1.

125. Collinson PO, Stubbs PJ, Rosalki SB. Cardiac troponin T in renal disease. Clin Chem 1995; 41:1671-3.

126. Cummins B, Auckland ML, Cummins P. Cardiac-specific troponin-I radioimmunoassay in the diagnosis of acute myocardial infarction. Am Heart J 1987; 113:1333-44.

127. Vallins WJ, Brand NJ, Dabjade N et al. Molecular cloning of human troponin I using polymerase chain reaction. FEBS Lett 1990; 270:57-61.

128. Saggin L, Gorza L, Ausoni S, Schiaffino S. Troponin I switching in the developing heart. J Biol Chem 1989; 264:16299-302.

129. Bhavsar P, Dhoot GK, Cumming DVE et al. Developmental expression of troponin I isoforms in fetal human heart. FEBS Lett 1991; 292:5-8.

130. Bodor GS, Porterfield D, Voss EM et al. Cardiac troponin I is not expressed in fetal and healthy and diseased adult human skeletal muscle tissue. Clin Chem 1995; 41:1710-5.

131. Martin AF. Turnover of cardiac troponin subunits. J Biol Chem 1981; 256:964-8.

132. Adams JE III, Schechtman KB, Landt Y et al. Comparable detection of acute myocardial infarction by creatine kinase MB isoenzyme and cardiac troponin I. Clin Chem 1994; 40:1291-5.

133. Cummins B, Cummins P. Cardiac specific troponin I release in canine experimental myocardial infarction: Development of a sensitive enzyme-linked immunoassay. J Mol Cell Cardiol 1987; 19:999-1010.

134. Mair J, Wagner I, Morass B et al. Cardiac troponin I release correlates with myocardial infarction size. Eur J Clin Chem Clin Biochem 1995; 33:869-72.

135. Larue C, Calzolari C, Bertinchant JP et al. Cardiac-specific immunoenzymometric assay of troponin I in the early phase of acute myocardial infarction. Clin Chem 1993; 39:972-9.

136. Mair J, Thome-Kromer B, Wagner I et al. Concentration time courses of troponin and myosin subunits after acute myocardial infarction. Coronary Artery Dis 1994; 5:865-72.

137. Stanton E, Jackowski G, Worron I et al. Biochemical differentiation between the different classes of unstable angina (abstract). The Journal of Heart Failure 1995; 2:A387.

138. Hunt AC, Chow SL, Shiu MF et al. Release of creatine kinase-MB and cardiac specific troponin-I following percutaneous transluminal coronary angioplasty. Eur Heart J 1991; 12:690-4.

139. Adams JE III, Sicard GA, Allen BT et al. Diagnosis of perioperative myocardial infarction with measurement of cardiac troponin I. New Engl J Med 1994; 330:670-4.

140. Mair J, Larue C, Mair P et al. Use of cardiac troponin I to diagnose perioperative myocardial infarction in coronary artery bypass grafting. Clin Chem 1994; 40:2066-70.

141. Etievent JP, Chocron S, Toubin G et al. Use of cardiac troponin I as a marker of perioperative myocardial ischemia. Ann Thorac Surg 1995; 59:1192-4.

142. Smith SC, Ladenson JH, Mason JW et al. Detection of myocarditis by cardiac troponin I (abstract). Circulation 1994; 90(suppl-I):547.

143. Grant JW, Canter CE, Spray TL et al. Elevated donor cardiac troponin I—a marker of acute graft failure in infant heart recipients. Circulation;1994; 90:2618-21.

144. Adams JE III, Davila-Roman VG, Bossey PQ et al. Improved detection of cardiac contusion with cardiac troponin I. Am Heart J

1996; 131: 308-12.

145. Adams JE III, Bodor GS, Davila-Roman VG et al. Cardiac troponin I—a marker with high specificity for cardiac injury. Circulation 1993; 88:101-6.

146. Trinquier S, Flecheux O, Bullenger M et al. Highly specific immunoassay for cardiac troponin I assessed in noninfarct patients with chronic renal failure or severe polytrauma (letter). Clin Chem 1995; 41:1676.

147. Diederich KW, Eisele I, Ried T et al. Isolation and characterization of the complete human beta-myosin heavy chain gene. Hum Genet 1989; 81:214-20.

148. Bredman JJ, Wessels A, Weijs WA et al. Demonstration of "cardiac-specific" myosin heavy chain in masticatory muscles of human and rabbit. Histochem J 1991; 23:160-70.

149. Bouvagnet P, Leger J, Pons F et al. Fiber types and myosin types in human atrial and ventricular myocardium. Circ Res 1984; 55:794-804.

150. Larue C, Calzolari C, Leger J et al. Immunoradiometric assay of myosin heavy chain fragments in plasma for investigation of myocardial infarction. Clin Chem 1991; 37:78-82.

151. Simeonova PP, Kehayov IR, Kyurkchiev SD. Identification of human ventricular myosin heavy chain fragments with monoclonal antibody 2F4 in human sera after myocardial necrosis. Clin Chim Acta 1991; 201:207-22.

152. Leger JOC, Larue C, Ming T et al. Assay of serum cardiac myosin heavy chain fragments in patients with acute myocardial infarction: determination of infarct size and long-term follow-up. Am Heart J 1990; 120:781-90.

153. Mair J, Wagner I, Jakob G et al. Different time courses of cardiac contractile proteins after acute myocardial infarction. Clin Chim Acta 1994; 231:47-60.

154. Seguin JR, Saussine M, Ferriere M et al. Myosin: a highly sensitive indicator of myocardial necrosis after cardiac operations. J Thorac Cardiovasc Surg 1989; 98:397-401.

155. Bandman E. Contractile protein isoforms in muscle development. Dev Biol 1992; 154:273-90.

156. Horvath BZ, Gaetjens E. Immunochemical studies on the light chains from skeletal muscle myosin. Biochim Biophys Acta 1972; 263:779-93.

157. Katus HA, Yasada T, Gold HK et al. Diagnosis of acute myocardial infarction by detection of circulating cardiac myosin light chains. Am J Cardiol 1984; 54:964-70.

158. Khaw BA, Gold HK, Fallon JT et al. Detection of serum cardiac myosin light chains in acute experimental myocardial infarction: radioimmunoassay of cardiac myosin light chains. Circulation 1978; 58:1130-6.

159. Gere JB, Krauth GH, Trahern CA et al. A radioimmunoassay for the measurement of human cardiac myosin light chains. Am J Clin Pathol 1979; 71:309-18.

160. Katus HA, Diederich KW, Uellner M et al. Myosin light chains release in acute myocardial infarction: non-invasive estimation of infarct size. Cardiovasc Res 1988; 22:456-63.

161. Wang J, Shi Q, Wu TW et al. The quantitation of human ventricular myosin light chain 1 in serum after myocardial necrosis and infarction. Clin Chim Acta 1989; 181:325-36.

162. Katus HA, Diederich KW, Schwarz F et al. Influence of reperfusion on serum concentrations of cytosolic creatine kinase and structural myosin light chains in acute myocardial infarction. Am J Cardiol 1987; 60:440-5.

163. Isobe M, Nagai R, Ueda S et al. Quantitative relationship between left ventricular function and serum cardiac myosin light chain I levels after coronary reperfusion in patients with acute myocardial infarction. Circulation 1987; 76:1251-61.

164. Nagai R, Chiu CC, Yamaoki K et al. Evaluation of methods for estimating infarct size by myosin LC2: comparison with cardiac enzymes. Am J Physiol 1983; 245:H413-9.

165. Mair J, Wagner I, Fridrich L et al. Cardiac myosin light chain-1 release in acute myocardial infarction is associated with scintigraphic estimates of myocardial scar. Clin Chim Acta 1994; 229:153-9.

166. Omura T, Teregaki M, Tagaki M et al. Myocardial infarct size by serum troponin T and myosin light chain-1 concentration. Jpn Circ J 1995; 59:154-9.

167. Uchino T, Belboul A, Roberts D et al. Measurement of myosin light chain 1 and troponin T as markers of myocardial cell damage after cardiac surgery. J Cardiovasc Surg 1994; 35:201-6.

168. Nakai K, Itoh C, Kikuchi M et al. Increased serum levels of human cardiac myosin light chain 1 in patients with renal failure. Rinsho Byori 1992; 40:529-34.

169. Fukunaga H, Higuchi I, Usuki F et al. Clinical significance of serum cardiac myosin light chain 1 in patients with Duchenne muscular dystrophy. No To Shinkei 1992; 44:131-5.

170. Mair J, Smidt J, Lechleitner P et al. A decision tree for the early diagnosis of acute myocardial infarction in nontraumatic chest pain patients at hospital admission. Chest 1995; 108:1502-9.

171. Newgard CB, Hwang PK, Fletterick RJ. The family of glycogen phosphorylases: structure and function. Crit Rev Biochem Molec Biol 1989; 24:69-99.

172. Meyer F, Heilmeyer LMG Jr, Haschke RH et al. Control of phosphorylase activity in a muscle glycogen particle: isolation and characterization of the protein-glycogen complex. J Biol Chem 1970; 245:6642-8.

173. Entman ML, Kaniike K, Goldstein MA et al. A. Association of

glycogenolysis with cardiac sarcoplasmic reticulum. J Biol Chem 1976; 251:3140-6.

174. Entman ML, Bornet EP, van Winkle WB et al. Association of glycogenolysis with cardiac sarcoplasmic reticulum: II. Effect of glycogen depletion, deoxycholate solubilization and cardiac ischemia: evidence for a phosphorylase kinase membrane complex. J Mol Cell Cardiol 1977; 9:515-28.

175. Newgard CB, Littmann DR, Genderen C et al. Human brain glycogen phosphorylase. Cloning sequence analysis, chromosomal mapping, tissue expression and comparison with the human liver and muscle isozymes. J Biol Chem 1988; 263:3850-7.

176. Kato A, Shimizu A, Kurobe N et al. Human brain-type glycogen phosphorylase: quantitative localization in human tissues determined with an immunoassay system. J Neurochem 1989; 52:1425-32.

177. Will H, Krause E-G, Böhm M et al. Kinetische Eigenschaften der Isoenzyme der Glykogenphosphorylase b aus Herz- und Skelettmuskulatur des Menschen. Acta Biol Med Germ 1974; 33:149-60.

178. Proux D, Dreyfus JC. Phosphorylase isoenzymes in tissues: prevalence of the liver type in man. Clin Chim Acta 1973; 48:167-72.

179. Dobson JG, Mayer SE. Mechanism of activation of cardiac glycogen phosphorylase in ischemia and anoxia. Circ Res 1973; 33:412-20.

180. Kalil-Filho R, Gersdtenblith G, Hansford RG et al. Regulation of myocardial glycogenolysis during post-ischemic reperfusion. J Mol Cell Cardiol 1991; 23:1467-79.

181. Michael LH, Hunt JR, Weilbaecher D et al. Creatine kinase and phosphorylase in cardiac lymph: coronary occlusion and reperfusion. Am J Physiol 1985; 248:H350-9.

182. Krause E-G, Will H, Böhm M et al. The assay of glycogen phosphorylase in human blood serum and its application to the diagnosis of myocardial infarction. Clin Chim Acta 1975; 58:145-54.

183. Schulze W, Krause E-G, Wollenberger A. On the fate of glycogen phosphorylase in the ischemic and infarcting myocardium. J Mol Cell Cardiol 1971; 2:241-51.

184. Krause E-G, Härtwig A, Rabitzsch G. On the release of glycogen phosphorylase from heart muscle: effect of substrate depletion, ischemia and of imipramine. Biomed Biochim Acta 1989; 48:S77-82.

185. Rabitzsch G, Mair J, Lechleitner P et al. Isoenzyme BB of glycogen phosphorylase b and myocardial infarction. Lancet 1993; 341:1032-3.

186. Rabitzsch G, Mair J, Lechleitner P et al. Immunoenzymometric assay of human glycogen phosphorylase isoenzyme BB in diagnosis of ischemic myocardial injury. Clin Chem 1995; 41:966-78.

187. Mair J, Puschendorf B, Smidt J et al. Early release of glycogen phosphorylase in patients with unstable angina and transient ST-T

alterations. Brit Heart J 1994; 72:125-7.

188. Mair P, Mair J, Krause E-G et al. Glycogen phosphorylase isoenzyme BB mass release after coronary artery bypass grafting. Eur J Clin Chem Clin Biochem 1994; 32:543-7.

189. Kleine AH, Glatz JFK, van Nieuwenhoven FA et al. Release of heart fatty acid-binding protein into plasma after acute myocardial infarction in man. Mol Cell Biochem 1992; 116:155-62.

190. Glatz JFC, van der Vusse GJ. Cellular fatty acid-binding proteins: current concepts and future directions. Mol Cell Biochem 1990; 98:237-51.

191. Roos W, Eymann E, Symannek M et al. Monoclonal antibodies to human heart fatty acid-binding protein. J Immunol Methods 1995; 183:149-53.

192. Ohkaru Y, Asayama K, Ishii H et al. Development of a sandwich enzyme-linked immunosorbent assay for the determination of human heart-type fatty acid-binding protein in plasma and urine by using two different monoclonal antibodies specific for human heart fatty acid-binding protein. J Immunol Methods 1995; 178:99-111.

193. Watanabe K, Wakabayashi H, Veerkamp JH et al. Immunohistochemical distribution of heart-type fatty acid binding protein immunoreactivity in normal human tissues and in acute myocardial infarct. J Pathol 1993; 170:59-65.

194. Kragten JA, van Nieuwenhoven FA, van Dieijen-Visser MP et al. Distribution of myoglobin and fatty acid binding protein in human heart. Clin Chem 1996; 42: 337-8.

195. Van Nieuwenhoven FA, Kleine AH, Wodzig KWH et al. Discrimination between myocardial and skeletal muscle injury by assessment of the plasma ratio of myoglobin over fatty acid binding protein. Circulation 1995; 92:2848-54.

196. Sohmiya K, Tanaka T, Tsuji R et al. Plasma and urinary heart-type cytoplasmic fatty acid-binding protein in coronary occlusion and reperfusion induced myocardial injury. J Mol Cell Cardiol 1993; 25:1413-26.

197. Glatz JFC, Kleine AH, van Nieuwenhoven FA et al. Fatty-acid binding protein as a plasma marker for the estimation of myocardial infarct size in humans. Br Heart J 1994; 71:135-40.

198. Tsuji R, Tanaka T, Sohmiya K et al. Human heart-type cytoplasmic fatty acid binding protein in serum and urine during hyperacute myocardial infarction. Int J Cardiol 1993; 41:209-17.

199. Jeffery S, Carter N, Edwards Y. Distribution of CA III in fetal and adult human tissue. Biochem Genet 1980; 18:843-9.

200. Sly WS, Hu PY. Human carbonic anhydrases and carbonic anhydrase deficiencies. Ann Rev Biochem 1995; 64:375-401.

201. Väänänen HK, Leppilampi M, Vuori J et al. Liberation of muscle carbonic anhydrase into serum during extensive exercise. J Appl Physiol 1986; 61:561-4.

202. Väänänen HK, Syrjälä H, Rahkila P et al. Serum carbonic anhydrase III and myoglobin concentrations in acute myocardial infarction. Clin Chem 1990; 36:635-8.
203. Brogan GX, Vuori J, Friedman S et al. Improved specificity of myoglobin plus carbonic anhydrase assay versus that of creatine kinase-MB for early diagnosis of acute myocardial infarction. Ann Emerg Med 1996; 27:22-8.
204. Vuori J, Syrjälä H, Väänänen HK. Myoglobin/carbonic anhydrase III ratio: highly specific and sensitive early indicator for myocardial damage in acute myocardial infarction. Clin Chem 1996; 42:107-9.
205. Uchida K, Kondoh K, Matuo Y. Recombinant M-, B-, and MB-type isozymes of human phosphoglyceric acid mutase: their large-scale production and preparation of polyclonal antibodies specific to M- and B-type isozymes. Clin Chim Acta 1995; 237:43-58.
206. Omenn GS, Cheung SCY. Phosphoglycerate mutase isozyme marker for tissue differentiation in man. Am J Hum Genet 1974; 26:393-9.
207. Yares S, Jeffery S, Barnard P et al. Plasma phosphoglycerate mutase muscle (M) isoenzyme is strikingly raised in Duchenne muscular dystrophy. Biochem Soc Trans 1986; 14:1165-6.
208. Kato K, Ishiguro Y, Ariyoshi Y. Enolase isoenzymes as disease markers: distribution of three enolase subunits (α, β, and γ) in variuos human tissues. Dis Markers 1983; 1:213-20.
209. Nomura M, Kato K, Nagasaka A et al. Serum β-enolase in acute myocardial infarction. Br Heart J 1987; 58:29-33.
210. Herraz-Dominguez M, Goldberg D, Anderson A et al. Serum enolase and pyruvate kinase activities in the diagnosis of myocardial infarction. Enzyme 1976; 21:211-24.
211. Usui A, Kato K, Abe T et al. β-enolase in blood plasma during open heart surgery. Cardiovasc Res 1989; 23:737-40.
212. van Landeghem AAJ, Soons JBJ, Wever RA et al. Purification and determination of the modifying protein responsible for the post-synthetic modification of creatine kinase and enolase. Clin Chim Acta 1985; 153:217-34.
213. Kato K, Kimura S, Haimoto H et al. S100a_0 ($\alpha\alpha$) protein: distribution in muscle tissues of various animals and purification from human pectoral muscle. J Neurochem 1986; 46:1555-60.
214. Kato K, Kimura S. S100a_0 protein is mainly located in the heart and striated muscles. Biochim Biophys Acta 1985; 842:146-50.
215. Usui A, Kato K, Sasa H et al. S-100a_0 protein in serum during acute myocardial infarction. Clin Chem 1990; 36:639-41.
216. Usui A, Kato K, Abe T et al. S-100 protein in blood and urine during open heart surgery. Clin Chem 1989; 35:1942-4.

CHAPTER 6

ACCUMULATED METABOLITES OF ISCHEMIC MYOCARDIUM:
UTILITY AS DIAGNOSTIC MARKERS

LACTATE

BACKGROUND

The human heart uses mainly fatty acids and also lactate as an energy substrate under normal conditions (lactate consumer). However, during ischemia also heart muscle switches to glucose as the main energy substrate. Glycogen is broken down, and during ischemia glucose is not completely metabolized, lactate accumulates within cardiomyocytes. Subsequently lactate is released from the cardiomyocytes, and the heart becomes a lactate producer.

USAGE OF LACTATE DETERMINATION AS A MARKER OF MYOCARDIAL ISCHEMIA IN CARDIOLOGY

Lactate is a classic parameter for the laboratory monitoring of ischemia or hypoxia. It can be quickly measured, either enzymatically or using lactate oxidase electrodes. Whole blood systems for bedside measurements are available for routine use. During severe myocardial ischemia (e.g., unstable angina, infarcting myocardium) the heart switches from lactate consumption to lactate production and release. However, lactate is produced by many tissues during hypoxia and ischemia. Therefore, measurement of blood lactate concentrations in the systemic circulation is unspecific, because the lactate levels are influenced by many factors. Systemic lactate measurements do not play an important role in the laboratory diagnosis of myocardial ischemia or infarction. However, blood lactate was a useful predictor for the development of cardiogenic shock in patients with acute myocardial infarction (AMI).[1] Left ventricular failure causes hypoxia of many tissues, which leads to an increase in systemic blood lactate concentrations.

However, if it is possible to measure lactate in coronary sinus venous blood samples, lactate is a very useful marker for the assessment of cardiac energy metabolism, for example in cardiac surgery.[2] The energy state of the human heart can be monitored intraoperatively before and during cardioplegia or during reperfusion and rewarming of the cardioplegic organ by means of the arterio-coronary venous difference in lactate concentrations. During ischemia coronary sinus lactate concentration increases significantly above the arterial concentration. Immediately after aortic unclamping with the restoration of coronary artery blood flow a transient increase in lactate of the coronary sinus blood is usually observed. This reflects the wash-out of the accumulated metabolite during cardioplegia and a rapidly re-established aerobic adenosine triphosphate (ATP) supply via oxidative phosphorylation in the mitochondria. A prolonged high lactate concentration in the coronary venous blood during reperfusion, on the other hand, indicates a delay in the normalization of aerobic ATP synthesis. This leads to a delayed re-establishment of the cardiac pump function, and catecholamine therapy is frequently needed in these patients. Metabolic monitoring by coronary sinus lactate measurements frequently allows to diagnose myocardial ischemia before its hemodynamic consequences can be firmly assessed by hemodynamic parameters or as wall motion abnormalities in echocardiography. Of course, a lactate monitoring is hampered or impossible if the solution used for cardioplegia is substituted by high concentrations of lactate.

Locally drawn blood samples in patients undergoing an exercise stress test with invasive hemodynamic monitoring (Swan-Ganz-catheter) may allow to detect myocardial ischemia also by lactate measurements.[2]

CREATINE
Creatine is another analyte which has been proposed for the early diagnosis of AMI. Creatine can be measured specifically by an enzymatic assay which is based on the use of creatinase, sarcosinoxidase, and peroxidase catalyzed reactions that form a dye.[3] This method is easily adaptable to autoanalyzers. The reaction time is only 8 minutes.

BIOCHEMISTRY

Creatine is a low-molecular-mass compound (MW 131 kDa) abundant in both skeletal muscle and myocardium.[4] Human heart contains about 2-3 mg creatine/g wet weight. After AMI, because of direct leakage of creatine from the infarcting myocardium, a transient increase in creatine concentrations in blood can be predicted. As a low molecular mass compound it should quickly appear in blood. Because of the existence of a renal threshold for creatine, creatinuria only occurs when serum concentrations exceed this value. The renal threshold is about 70 μmol/L, which is slightly above the physiological serum concentrations.[3]

The daily needs for creatine are covered by endogenous synthesis. Creatine is synthesized in two steps: (1) in the kidneys guanidino-acetic acid is synthesized from arginine and glycine and (2) in the liver guanidino-acetic acid is methylated to creatine.[4] Creatine is secreted into the blood, and it is taken up by heart and skeletal muscle fibers by an active transport mechanism. In the muscle 70% is found as creatine phosphate and 30% as creatine.[4] Creatine phosphate is an important energy storage within muscle fibers (45 kJ/mol).[4]

When comparing serum creatine and cardiac protein concentrations, one should consider that the metabolism of creatine is entirely different from the metabolism of cardiac proteins:[5] (1) creatine is not synthesized in the heart; (2) its molecular mass is much lower than that of cardiac proteins; (3) creatine is kept in viable myocytes, due to an active pump mechanism; (4) extracellular creatine is actively taken up by viable muscle fibers; (5) creatine is found in the glomerular filtrate. In the kidney tubuli, there is an active reuptake process for the creatine present in the glomerular filtrate, which is characterized by a renal threshold value and (6) creatine and creatine phosphate are spontaneously metabolized into creatinine at a constant rate.

CLINICAL RESULTS

Acute myocardial infarction

In the acute phase of AMI (2-8 hours after onset of symptoms) an early transient increase in the creatine concentration in serum and urine can be observed.[3] However increased concentrations were only found in about 70% of the investigated AMI patients because of a considerable overlap of controls and AMI patients. Increases were missing, particularly in small AMIs. Peak concentrations in plasma are observed about 2-4 hours after the onset of chest pain with a rapid decrease thereafter. The biological half-life is about 1-2 hours. Serum creatine determinations are not useful 6 hours after chest pain onset or later. Due to the renal threshold, determination of urine values in the first urine sample after chest pain onset gives a better discrimination between infarction patients and controls than does serum determination.[3] In urine samples peaks are reached approximately 60 minutes after the serum peak.[3] The levels rapidly return to normal within 1-3 hours after maximal concentrations. Because of the urine storage capacity of the bladder, the urinary creatine stays elevated for a longer time period than serum creatine. Creatine values are not closely correlated with infarct size. Creatine leakage from myocardium is deemed to be insufficient to explain the observed creatinuria in AMI patients, and intact extra-cardiac tissues are believed to be involved in creatine release,[3,5] because the predicted changes from postmortem creatine losses from the infarcted zone are much smaller. Increased de novo sythesis is insufficient to produce such large quantities of creatine in a short period of time.[3] In about 40% of AMI patients secondary peaks of serum and urine creatine concentrations can be seen about 24-36 hours after hospital admissions which are not explained by recurrent AMI. The reason for this biphasic behavior is not known so far, because no correlation could be observed between the occurrence of secondary creatine peaks and the clinical situation of the patient.[5] Thrombolytic therapy neither significantly influenced time-to-peak values nor maximal creatine concentrations in serum.[5]

Unstable angina pectoris

Serum and urine creatine levels after an acute episode of chest pain showed no significant changes.[3,5]

Cardiac surgery

In patients undergoing cardiac surgery changes in serum creatine concentration were small, despite the presence of muscle trauma. Peak values did not differ significantly from controls.[5]

SPECIFICITY OF CREATINE

Creatine is not a heart-specific marker, it is abundant in heart and skeletal muscle. The creatine content of other tissues is too low so that damage usually does not increase serum or urinary creatine. However, increased creatine was observed in patients with hyper- or hypothyreosis.[5] Influence of creatine-containing diet on creatine concentrations in serum and urine is limited, as creatine is absorbed very rapidly after ingestion and the plasma half-life is short.[5]

The major source of false positive results is skeletal muscle. For example intramuscular injections of 5 ml saline solution (0.9%) and muscular trauma due to other causes (e.g., exercise, trauma, surgery) lead to an increase of creatine in blood and urine. Intramuscular injections of 5 ml revealed a marked increase in serum creatine after a period of 1 hours, and also increases in urine creatine were observed afterwards.[3,5] Injections of only 2 ml led to only mild increases.

CLINICAL USEFULNESS OF CREATINE DETERMINATIONS

Thus far creatine measurements were only compared with CK and CKMB activity measurements which are known to lack sensitivity during the early phase of AMI. Comparisons with more sensitive markers, such as myoglobin and CKMB mass or CK isoforms, are missing. A major limitation of creatine is that the sensitivity for AMI is below 100%, that is in some AMI patients, particularly with small infarctions, creatine never exceeded the upper reference limit in serial samples.[3,5] In contrast to proteins, excess creatine can be taken up by still viable muscle fibers by an active pump mechanism.[4] Therefore, absence of an increase in serum creatine concentration means that the net difference between the rate of creatine release and the rate of active uptake is small. This, however, excludes the clinically more important detection of minor myocardial injury in patients with unstable angina. Even small AMIs may be missed.

From its tissue distribution it can be derived that creatine is not a heart-specific marker. The diagnostic specificity has not been tested in unselected patients so far. Renal failure will increase serum creatine (false positive results) as this molecule is also eliminated from blood by the kidneys. On the other hand, dietary creatine intake also affects creatine plasma concentrations, and high dietary intake of creatine, for example by athletes, may lead to transient false positive results.

In summary, because of its limited sensitivity, particularly for minor myocardial injury and small AMIs, and its lack of cardiac specificity, creatine is not an important marker for the early diagnosis of myocardial injury and will not play a major role in the diagnosis of myocardial damage in the future, because more suitable markers are available.

ADENOSINE, INOSINE, HYPOXANTHINE, AND XANTHINE

BIOCHEMISTRY

In the hypoxic cardiomyocyte, adenosine triphosphate (ATP) strongly decreases and the content of adenosine monophosphate (AMP) increases to the same extent. Subsequently, adenosine, inosine, and hypoxanthine are formed from AMP, and these metabolites accumulate and are released (see chapter 7). If blood flow is restored hypoxanthine is metabolized to xanthine and in a second step to uric acid.

CLINICAL RESULTS

Increases in all four parameters have been described in AMI patients or in coronary sinus blood samples of patients undergoing coronary artery bypass grafting.[6-8] A delayed increase in hypoxanthine and xanthine was observed in systemic blood samples after AMI.[6] Hypoxanthine increases were found on average only after 7.7 ± 4.2 hours and xanthine increases 9.8 ± 5.9 hours after chest pain onset.[6] The sensitivities and specificities of all four parameters were limited. These analytes are formed in every ischemic tissue. The delayed increase of hypoxanthine and xanthine suggests that they are not mainly released from the myocardium, because in this case increases and peaks are expected to occur earlier (see, e.g., creatine). It is likely that inflammatory cells which enter the infarcted myocardium contribute to the observed increases in both analytes.

Moreover, adenosine, inosine, hypoxanthine and xanthine can be only accurately measured using high pressure liquid chromatography (HPLC). Mistakes in the preanalytical phase (e.g., hemolysis) may influence hypoxanthine results. For these reasons and because of their limited diagnostic sensitivities and specificities for AMI these accumulated metabolites are not analytes for routine use. Their application will be restricted to investigations on the pathophysiology of myocardial infarction and reperfusion injury.

REFERENCES

1. Mavric Z, Zaputovic L, Zagar D et al. Usefulness of blood lactate as a predictor of shock development in acute myocardial infarction. Am J Cardiol 1991; 67:565-8.

2. Krause EG, Pfeiffer D, Wollenberger U et al. Application of the lactate biosensor for the assessment of cardiac energy metabolism. In: Piper HM, Preusse CJ, eds. Ischemia-Reperfusion in Cardiac Surgery. Dodrecht-Boston-London: Kluver Academic Publishers, 1993:328-33.

3. Delanghe J, De Buyzere M, De Scheerder I et al. Creatine determinations as an early marker for the diagnosis of acute myocardial infarction. Ann Clin Biochem 1988; 25:383-8.

4. Walker J. Creatine: biosynthesis, regulation, and function. Adv Enzymol 1980; 48:177-242.

5. Delanghe JR, De Buyzere ML, Scheerder IKD et al. Characteristics of creatine release during acute myocardial infarction, unstable angina, and cardiac surgery. Clin Chem 1995; 41:928-33.

6. Kock R, Delvoux B, Sigmund M et al. A comparative study of the concentrations of hypoxanthine, xanthine, uric acid and allantoin in peripheral blood of normals and patients with acute myocardial infarction and other ischemic diseases. Eur J Clin Chem Clin Biochem 1994; 32:837-42.

7. Giardina B, Penco M, Lazzarino G et al. Effectiveness of thrombolysis is associated with a time dependent increase of malondialdehyde in peripheral blood of patients with acute myocardial infarction. Am J Cardiol 1993; 71:788-93.

8. Kaukinen S, Metsa-Ketela T, Kaukinen L et al. Biochemical indicators of myocardial ischemia during coronary artery bypass grafting. Scand J Thorac Cardiovasc Surg 1990; 24:71-3.

CHAPTER 7

PATHOPHYSIOLOGICAL BASIS OF PROTEIN RELEASE AFTER MYOCARDIAL DAMAGE

MECHANISMS OF INTRAMYOCARDIAL PROTEIN RELEASE IN MYOCARDIAL DAMAGE

Cellular injury can be caused by chemical, microbial, and physical agents, and deprivation of normal nutritional requirements, e.g., anoxia or ischemia. Most types of cell death are delayed with a substantial reversible prelethal phase.

DEVELOPMENT OF CELL INJURY IN SUSTAINED ACUTE MYOCARDIAL ISCHEMIA

Myocardial ischemia is present whenever the coronary arterial flow cannot provide enough oxygen to meet the demands of myocardium. The extent of ischemia after occlusion of a coronary artery depends on the presence of preformed collateral anastomoses. Sudden induction of myocardial ischemia by occlusion of a major branch of a coronary artery in human heart sets into motion a series of events that culminates in death of markedly ischemic myocytes (reviewed in refs. 1, 2). These alterations include cessation of contraction, ECG changes, and onset of anaerobic glycolysis and appear simultaneously. If ischemia persists, many affected myocytes become irreversibly injured. Brief periods of ischemia ($\leq$15 minutes) are tolerated and myocytes will recover. Most severely ischemic myocytes (subendocardial region) are dead in regional ischemia in the anesthetized open-chest dog heart after only

60 minutes of ischemia. Less severely ischemic myocytes in the mid- and subepicardial myocardium survive for as long as six hours. Virtually all myocytes are irreversibly injured after six hours of ischemia have passed.[2] Ions (e.g., potassium) leak from damaged cardiomyocytes within seconds, metabolites (e.g., lactate, adenosine, inosine) within minutes, and macromolecules (e.g., cardiac cytoplasmatic enzymes) within hours.

These changes initiated by myocardial ischemia begin within seconds of occlusion and include:

1. cessation of aerobic metabolism;
2. depletion of creatine phosphate;
3. onset of anaerobic glycolysis;
4. accumulation of products of anaerobic metabolism in ischemic tissue.

Within seconds from the onset of ischemia the oxygen present in capillaries (oxyhemoglobin) and myocytes (oxymyoglobin) is exhausted. The myocardium ceases contracting, converts to anaerobic metabolism, and develops electrophysiological changes (membrane potential begins to decrease, ECG changes appear). Reserves of high energy phosphates in myocardium are quite small. In the dog heart, enough adenosine triphosphate (ATP) or creatine phosphate available to support only three or four efficient beats.[2] Myocardium converts to anaerobic glycolysis as its chief means of generating new high-energy phosphate. The ATP demands are immediately tried to be reduced by depressed contractile activity, which leads to wall motion abnormalities in, e.g., echocardiography. Glycogen stores are metabolized to lactate. Within 1-2 minutes anaerobic glycolysis slows down due to inhibition of glyceraldehyde phosphate dehydrogenase by high cytosolic reduced nicotinamide adenine dinucleotide adenine dinucleotide ratio (NADH/NAD$^+$), low pH, and high lactate levels. Glycolysis persists at a slower rate for about 1 hour and then ceases. The exact cause of the cessation of glycolysis early in the phase of irreversible injury is not known. It is likely that it is due to low sarcoplasmatic ATP and/or allosteric and end-product inhibitions of various glycolytic reactions. Creatine phosphate, which is the main reserve source of high-energy phosphates in myocardium, is used within seconds of occlusion to rephosphorylate adenosine diphosphate (ADP). This reaction is catalyzed by creatine kinase. Anaerobic glycolysis also cannot sufficiently provide ATP. As a consequence tissue ADP increases, adenylate kinase is activated and forms from two ADP one ATP with one adenosine monophosphate (AMP). AMP accumulates, and excess AMP is progressively dephosphorylated to adenosine. Adenosine is converted by adenosine deaminase to inosine. In contrast to AMP, inosine and adenosine can diffuse out of the cardiomyocyte into the interstitial space where they are further degraded to hypoxanthine and later also to xanthine. Human heart contains very little xanthine oxidase, and very little xanthine is formed during ischemia.

The accumulation of osmotically active particles arising from ischemic metabolism within cardiomyocytes (inorganic phosphate, protons, creatine, glycolytic intermediates, and catabolites of the adenine nucleotide pool) creates an osmotic load. The osmotic load begins to develop within seconds, and water enters the myocyte as a consequence of this. There is also an immediate efflux of potassium. This leads to a localized hyperpolarization, which leads to the typical ECG pattern of acute myocardial ischemia. Deregulation of cellular ionic homeostasis constitutes an important and early feature of cell injury. Increases in intracellular calcium also occur which result from increased influx and redistribution from intracellular compartments (endoplasmatic reticulum, mitochondria). Increasing intracellular calcium activates phospholipases, endonucleases, or the soluble protease calpain. Among myofibrillar proteins troponin T and troponin I are particularly susceptible to calpain digestion,[4] which may contribute to the early degradation, dissociation and release of these troponin subunits after myocardial damage (see troponin T and troponin I). The lysosomes are stable within the first 3-4 hours after onset of ischemia. Their proteolytic enzymes are, therefore, not causally related to the disintegration of myofilaments during the early stages of ischemic myocardial injury. pH dependent dissociation of the troponin complex could be another important factor for the early troponin release, apart from the presence of soluble precursor protein pools (see troponin I and troponin T).

Early ultrastructural changes in the reversible phase of ischemia include edema (e.g., swelling of sarcoplasmatic reticulum), condensed and later swollen mitochondria, disappearance of glycogen granules, and the nuclear chromatin begins to be aggregated peripherally (chromatin condensation). Cytoplasmic blebbing is also deemed to be possible in the reversible phase of cell injury.[3] The cytoplasmatic blebs may detach and the plasma membrane reseals without cell death.

Early in the irreversible phase of ischemic injury tissue is characterized by:

1. very low content of energy-rich phosphates (creatine phosphate <1-2% and ATP <10% of control);
2. a depressed adenine nucleotide pool that consists principally of AMP;
3. virtual cessation of anaerobic glycolysis;
4. low pH and low glycogen content;
5. high inosine and hypoxanthine contents;
6. a markedly increased osmolar load consisting chiefly of lactate;
7. characteristic ultrastructural changes.

These ultrastructural changes include cell swelling and evidence of generalized mitochondrial (disorganized cristae, amorphous densities in the matrix space) and marked sarcolemmal damage. Sarcolemmal disruption is believed to indicate morphologically the "point of no return". Contracture-rigor develops due to the presence of high levels of intracellular calcium. The so-called N-band also appears, which is not found in healthy tissue. Once the breaks develop in the plasmalemma, myocytes rapidly release intracellular macromolecules and gain high amounts of extracellular electrolytes, such as sodium and calcium, through these defects. Currently, it is believed that membrane disruption is a two-stage phenomenon.[1,2] First lesions of the attachment complex which includes vinculin, talin, integrin, and α-actin induced by ischemia must develop, and second, a force, such as cell swelling or contraction (contraction band formation), must disrupt the sarcolemma. Disruptions frequently begin to occur in the area of blebs. ATP depletion probably contributes to plasma membrane disruption and is a potential general cause of irreversibility of ischemic myocardial injury. Later on the classical morphological signs of infarction appear—loss of the nuclei and striation pattern of cardiomyocytes.

IS THE RELEASE OF INTRAMYOCARDIAL PROTEINS ALWAYS AN INDICATOR OF IRREVERSIBLE MYOCARDIAL INJURY?

This important question is still controversially discussed and a matter of debate. There are two hypotheses:[5]

1. The physiological impermeability of the sarcolemma for macromolecules (e.g., proteins) is a fixed property of the plasma membrane, and protein release from the cardiomyocyte is only possible from irreversible injured cardiomyocytes.
2. The physiological impermeability is a metabolically controlled property of the cell membrane. Extracellular rise of myocardial proteins may also follow in smaller amounts to reversible disturbances of cell metabolism.

The latter hypothesis seems to be confirmed by the results of some recent experimental and clinical studies. At moderate ischemic stress myocardial tissue can release small amounts of macromolecules from the cytosolic compartment by mechanical mechanisms other than persistent membrane perforation.[5-7] There is a relation between energy metabolism and enzyme release in cardiomyocytes.[5] Prevention of leakiness is directly or indirectly an energy consuming process. Myocardial plasma membranes become permeable for intracellular proteins if cells come into an energy-deficient state. Concentration gradient and spatial dimension of a protein strongly influence the correlation of its release and cellular energy state.[5] Piper et al[6] demonstrated that enzyme release into the medium was possible from reversibly injured cultured adult rat cardiomyocytes. Coronary occlusion in the dog or baboon of 15 minute duration caused a release of CK and glycogen phosphorylase without the development of histological signs of myocardial necrosis in the affected region of the myocardium.[8,9] Recently Remppis et al[10] reported a significant release of CK, LDH, and cardiac troponin T (cTnT) after 20 minutes of no flow ischemia, which rendered mitochondrial membranes intact and where electron dense bodies were found only occasionally. Experimental myocardial stress similar to diagnostic procedures of clinical routine may lead to myocardial enzyme release without histological evidence for myocardial necrosis development.[11] In clinical studies increases in CK and CK isoforms were found in coronary sinus venous blood after PTCA-induced coronary artery occlusion of not longer than 1 minute duration and after pacing induced myocardial ischemia in patients with coronary artery disease.[12,13] Myocardial necrosis as a source of protein release is very unlikely in these patient groups.

In summary, it seems to be possible that reversibly injured myocardium releases small amounts of soluble cytoplasmatic proteins (including the soluble troponin and myosin light chain pools) probably due to detachment of blebs and resealing of the plasma membrane (see above). But this is still controversial, because many researchers believe that even small releases of intracellular myocardial proteins are an indication of cell necrosis and that the current histological or radiologic techniques are just not sensitive enough to detect the cell necrosis when it is patchy and involves small numbers of cells. The relation between cellular protein leakage and cell death or the equivalence of enzymatic and histological estimates of infarct size has now been debated for many years, but no final answers were obtained. Less controversial and usually generally accepted is that the appearance of mitochondrial enzymes, such as mitochondrial CK, mitochondrial ASAT or glutamate dehydrogenase, in serum and prolonged increases (more than 2 days) in cardiac contractile and regulatory proteins indicate myocardial necrosis.

CARDIAC PROTEINS: THE ROUTE FROM HEART TO PLASMA

The transport of enzymes and proteins from heart to plasma has been reviewed by Spiekermann et al.[14] Newer aspects were discussed by Van Kreel et al.[15] According to current knowledge all myocardial marker proteins appear in the interstitial space more or less at the same time. cTnT increased in parallel to CK and LDH after global ischemia and calcium paradox or reoxygenation.[10,16] We found a simultaneous release of cardiac troponin I (cTnI), cTnT, LDH, and CK from isolated perfused Langendorff rat hearts during reoxygenation after 60 minutes of hypoxia.[17] This could be confirmed in cultured adult rat cardiomyocytes in a model of hypoxia and reoxygenation (see Fig. 7.1). Vork et al found that fatty acid binding protein is released in parallel to LDH (a much larger molecule) from isolated rat hearts during normoxia, low-flow ischemia, and reperfusion.[18] During reperfusion after no-flow ischemia different release kinetics were found for cytosolic enzymes and cTnT.[10,16] Over the entire period of reperfusion cTnT concentrations increased in effluents, while cardiac enzyme activities rapidly declined at the end of reperfusion. The continuing release of cTnT must recruit from another intracellular compartment, i.e., the disintegrating contractile apparatus, indicating a loss of structural integrity.

Several studies showed that about 80% of the protein transport from heart to the general circulation occurs by direct entry of proteins into the microvessels.[14,15,19] The residual collateral flow (about 1% of normal conditions) is sufficient to flush the ischemic area every few minutes.[15] Some local retrograde venous flow could also stimulate this wash-out process. Even in the central infarcted area some residual flow remains present.[15] Therefore, the transport of proteins from the ischemic heart is not flow-limited. The remaining approximately 20% of protein transport is affected by lymph. As the heart is constantly beating, this transport is also relatively fast, and enzymes and proteins pass in about 20 minutes from the heart to the right lymphatic duct, which empties into

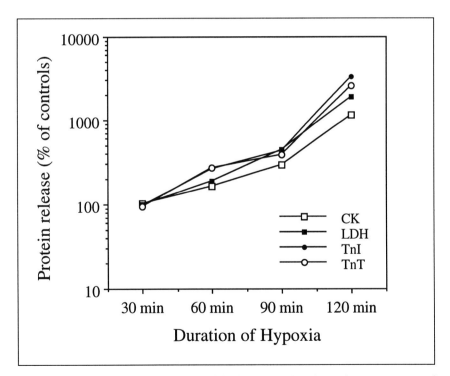

Fig. 7.1. Creatine kinase (CK), lactate dehydrogenase (LDH), cardiac troponin I and troponin T (TnI, TnT) release from cultured adult rat cardiomyocytes in a model of hypoxia and reoxygenation. Cardiomyocytes were cultured according to Piper et al[6] with slight modifications. The extent of marker release during reoxygenation is dependent on the duration of the preceding hypoxia. All markers increase in parallel. 30 minutes of hypoxia followed by reoxygenation does not lead to an enhanced protein release compared with controls. Data given as mean of four experiments.

the external jugular vein.[15] Thus, that minor fraction of proteins transported by lymph will also rapidly reach plasma.

Hydrophilic molecules (e.g., proteins) can cross capillaries of the heart by "pores" under normal conditions. Heart is a tissue with high capillary permeability. The endothelial cells are separated in the heart by small gaps (intercellular clefts). Small molecules are thought to pass the capillary walls through this "small-pore transport system". In addition, there are numerous pinocytotic vesicles within endothelial cells ("large-pore system") that are thought to be responsible for the transcapillary transport of large molecules, such as proteins. This system is more abundant in the walls of venous capillaries. Compared with skeletal muscle the density of capillaries in the heart is much higher, which results in a large area for direct entry into the microvessels by diffusion or pinocytosis. The capillaries are affected by ischemia as well. This includes separation of gap junctions, which modifies transcapillary transport properties. The protein permeability of the endothelial cell barrier increases by a factor of 2-3.[18,20] This further facilitates the direct entry of proteins into the capillaries and also stimulates lymph flow.

Reperfusion causes a true acceleration of cellular protein leakage and not just an enhanced wash-out.[15] This indicates an acute manifestation of plasmalemmal disruption but not necessarily implies the existence of "reperfusion injury", because the proteins could originate from cells that were already injured irreversibly at the time of reperfusion. In this case, reperfusion only made this injury manifest. The cardiomyocytes would also have leaked their enzymes without it, but more slowly.

FACTORS INFLUENCING THE FIRST APPEARANCE AND TIME COURSES OF A MARKER PROTEIN IN THE GENERAL CIRCULATION

INTRACELLULAR COMPARTMENTALIZATION OF PROTEINS

The intracellular compartmentalization of a molecule has a great impact on the rapidity with which it is released after myocardial damage.[21] Myocardial ischemia interrupts metabolic pathways and subsequently reduces or inhibits intracellular energy production, which leads to a disturbed membrane permeability (see above). The consequence is a release of intracellular macromolecules. Cytosolic proteins are released more rapidly than structural proteins after damage of the sarcolemma. In contrast to the release of cytosolic proteins, where only membrane leakage is required in principal, the release of the structurally bound pool of contractile proteins requires both a leaky plasma membrane and a dissociation and/or degradation of the subcellular contractile apparatus, which is a timely slower process. Significant differences in the patterns of appearance in blood of myoglobin, myosin light chain-1 (MLC-1), cTnI, and cTnT which are molecules of grossly comparable molecular sizes (17800, 26000, 24000 and 37000 Da, respectively) were found.[21] On the other hand, CKMB a molecule of much higher molecular weight (86000 Da) increased somewhat earlier than cTnT, cTnI, and significantly earlier than MLC-1 after AMI. These differences in first appearance can be explained by the different cellular localization of these molecules. Myoglobin is a cytosolic protein and CK is predominantly located in the sarcoplasma of cardiomyocytes. cTnT and cTnI appeared before cMLC-1, which can be at least partly explained by larger cytosolic troponin pools. Approximately 1% of the total MLC content exists as a soluble cytosolic precursor pool for myosin synthesis in the myocardium, and on an absolute weight basis the cytosolic pool of TnT is approximately 50 times larger compared with MLC-1.[22] The percentage of the soluble cTnI pool is similar to that of the cytosolic cTnT precursor pool (i.e., approximately 5% of total cTnT or cTnI content).

These cytosolic pools account for the biphasic release kinetics of cTnI, cTnT and cMLC-1 after AMI.[21] The initial increase is probably from the soluble pool in the myocyte, while prolonged increase is from proteolytic degradation or pH dissociation of the myofilaments. This early release of troponin subunits could be the result not only of the presence of cTnI and cTnT in the sarcoplasma not incorporated into the myofibrils, but also from a rapid dissociation and degradation of the troponin complex and its constituents, which has been described during total global ischemia in rat and human hearts.[23,24] This could involve the activation of the sarcoplasmatic protease calpain (see above). In particular, the time course of cTnI after AMI suggests a rapid dissociation and/or degradation of the cTnI from the troponin complex, because cTnI release resembles that of CK. cTnI peaks in parallel to CK, but it stays increased for several days longer than CK.

Myosin heavy chains (MHC) are the latest marker to appear in the general circulation after AMI. We found no evidence for the existence of soluble cytosolic MHC. On the other hand, MHC is very resistant to proteolysis because of its central location in the myosin molecule and the thick filament, respectively. Mitochondrial enzymes are also released at a later stage of a pathological process and less than those of the cytoplasmatic compartment.

MOLECULAR WEIGHT

Current clinical as well as experimental results suggest that the molecular weight seems to be of minor importance for the pattern of appearance of a myocardial protein in blood after AMI compared with its cellular localization. It appears, that the impact of the molecular weight has been overestimated and overemphasized for many years. For example, CKMB is predominately located in the sarcoplasma. Its molecular weight is about 3.5 times that of MLC-1. Nevertheless, after AMI CKMB mass increases significantly earlier than MLC-1.[21] However, within the family of molecules with a certain intracellular compartmentalization the molecular weight is a determining factor in the release and appearance in blood after AMI, because heavier molecules diffuse at a slower rate, and particularly smaller molecules, such as myoglobin, may enter the vascular system to an even larger extent directly via the microvascular endothelium.

CONCENTRATION GRADIENT BETWEEN CARDIOMYOCYTES AND THE INTERSTITIAL SPACE

The higher the concentration differences of a marker between the cardiomyocytes and the interstitial space, the faster a parameter will translocate from sarcoplasma to the interstitial space as soon as the plasma membrane permeability is increased.

LOCAL BLOOD AND LYMPH FLOW

Another factor that affects the appearance of markers in the general circulation is local blood and lymphatic flow (see above). Early reperfusion of the infarct-related artery qualitatively upsets the release kinetics of cytosolic proteins and contractile proteins with considerable cytosolic precursor pools, such as cTnI and cTnT, due to accelerated release of proteins from the infarcted cardiomyocytes and also due to the so-called "wash-out phenomenon" of extracellular proteins (see above). By contrast, the release kinetics of MLC-1 and MHC after AMI are not significantly affected by early reperfusion. These proteins only have a small or no soluble cytoplasmatic precursor pool (see above).

ELIMINATION OF RELEASED MYOCARDIAL PROTEINS FROM BLOOD

Marker protein time courses after myocardial damage are also markedly influenced by their disappearance rate from blood. For example, the differences in the LDH and CK time courses in the subacute phase of AMI are explained not by differences in release, instead different biological half-life times are responsible (CK: approximately 10-15 hours; LDH-1 isoenzyme: about 4 days). The site and mechanism of removal of proteins from the circulation have not yet been fully elucidated. Most proteins appear to be catabolized. In general, proteins are metabolized in organs with a high metabolic rate, such as liver, pancreas, kidneys and the reticuloendothelial system. Smaller molecules, such as myoglobin and heart fatty acid binding protein, pass the glomerular membranes and can be found in the glomerular filtrate. These proteins are reabsorbed and subsequently metabolized in tubular epithelial cells of the kidneys. Therefore, impaired clearance from blood (e.g., renal or hepatic failure, hypothyroidism) also leads to prolonged marker increases. On the other hand, in patients with hypermetabolic states, such as hyperthyroidism, proteins may be more quickly metabolized and may decrease more rapidly than in other patients.

REFERENCES

1. Jennings RB, Murry CE, Steenbergen C et al. Development of cell injury in sustained acute ischemia. Circulation 1990; 82(suppl II):II-2-II-12.
2. Jennings RB, Reimer KA. The cell biology of acute myocardial ischemia. Annu Rev Med 1991; 42:225-46.
3. Trump BF, Berezesky IK. Calcium-mediated cell injury and cell death. FASEB J;1995; 9:219-28.
4. De Lisa F, De Tullio R, Salamino F et al. Specific degradation of troponin T and I by μ-calpain and its modulation by substrate phosphorylation. Biochem J 1995; 308:57-61.
5. Gebhard MM, Denkhaus, H, Sakai K et al. Energy metabolism and enzyme release. J Mol Med 1977; 2:271-83.
6. Piper HM, Schwartz P, Spahr R et al. Early enzyme release from myocardial cells is not due to irreversible cell damage. J Mol Cell

Cardiol 1984; 16:385-8.

7. Wienen W, Kammermeier H. Intra- and extracellular markers in interstitial transsudate of perfused rat hearts. Am J Physiol 1988; 254:H785-94.

8. Heyndrickx GR, Amano J, Kenna T et al. Creatine kinase release not associated with myocardial necrosis after short periods of coronary artery occlusion in conscious baboons. J Am Coll Cardiol 1985; 6:1299-1305.

9. Michael LH, Hunt JR, Weilbach D. Creatine kinase and phosphorylase in cardiac lymph: coronary occlusion and reperfusion. Am J Physiol 1985; 248:350-9.

10. Remppis A, Scheffold T, Greten J et al. Intracellular compartmentation of troponin T: release kinetics after global ischemia and calcium paradox in the isolated perfused rat heart. J Mol Cell Cardiol 1995; 27:793-803.

11. Nordbeck H, Kahles H, Preusse CJ et al. Enzymes in cardiac lymph and coronary blood under normal and pathophysiological conditions. J Mol Med 1977; 2:255-63.

12. Schofer J, Lampe F, Mathey DG et al. Increase of creatine kinase and creatine kinase MM-isoforms following successful and uncomplicated coronary angioplasty. Z Kardiol 1992; 81:326-30.

13. Chiong MA, Parker JO. Myocardial balance of inorganic phosphate and enzymes in man. Effects of tachykardia and ischemia. Circulation 1974; 49:283-90.

14. Spiekermann PG, Nordbeck H, Preusse CJ. From Heart to Plasma. In: Hearse DJ, De Leiris J, eds. Enzymes in Cardiology: Diagnosis and Research. New York: John Wiley, 1979:59-79.

15. Van Kreel B, Van der Veen, FH, Willems GM et al. Circulatory models in assessment of cardiac enzyme release in dogs. Am J Physiol 1993; 264:H747-54.

16. Asayama J, Yamahara Y, Ohta B et al. Release kinetics of cardiac troponin T in coronary effluent from isolated rat hearts during hypoxia and reoxygenation. Basic Res Cardiol 1992; 87:428-36.

17. Vorderwinkler KP, Mair J, Puschendorf B et al. Cardiac troponin I increases in parallel to cardiac troponin T, creatine kinase and lactate dehydrogenase in effluents from isolated perfused rat hearts after hypoxia-reoxygenation-induced myocardial injury. Clin Chim Acta 1996 1996; 251: 113-17.

18. Vork MM, Glatz JF, Surtel DA et al. Release of fatty acid binding protein and lactate dehydrogenase from isolated rat heart during normoxia, low-flow ischemia, and reperfusion. Can J Physiol Pharmacol 1993; 71:952-8

19. Sunnergreen KP, Rovetto MJ. Microvascular permeability characteristics of isolated perfused ischemic rat heart. J Mol Cell Cardiol 1980; 12:1011-31.

20. Dauber IM, VanBenthuysen KM, McMurty IF et al. Functional

coronary microvascular injury evident as increased permeability due to brief ischemia and reperfusion. Circ Res 1990; 66:986-98.

21. Mair J, Thome-Kromer B, Wagner I et al. Concentration time courses of troponin and myosin subunits after acute myocardial infarction. Coronary Artery Dis 1994; 5:865-72.

22. Katus HA, Remppis A, Scheffold T et al. Intracellular compartmentation of cardiac troponin T and its release kinetics in patients with reperfused and nonreperfused myocardial infarction. Am J Cardiol 1991; 67:1360-67.

23. Westfall MV, Solaro RJ. Alterations in myofibrillar function and protein profiles after complete global ischemia in rat hearts. Circ Res 1992; 70:302-13.

24. Hein S, Scheffold T, Schaper J. Ischaemia induces early changes to cytoskeletal and contractile proteins in diseased human myocardium. J Thorac Cardiovasc Surg 1995; 110:89-98.

CHAPTER 8

BIOCHEMICAL MARKERS AS DIAGNOSTIC UTILITIES IN PARTICULAR CLINICAL SETTINGS:

RECOMMENDATIONS FOR THE USE OF CURRENTLY COMMERCIALLY AVAILABLE BIOCHEMICAL MARKERS IN CLINICAL PRACTICE

The continuing search for the perfect biochemical marker of acute myocardial infarction (AMI) which is 100% sensitive and 100% specific at all times after onset of AMI will fail. The characteristics of biochemical markers for AMI are summarized in Table 8.1. Currently no single marker meets all the criteria of an ideal biochemical marker for the laboratory diagnosis of myocardial injury, but cardiac troponin T (cTnT) and in particular cardiac troponin I (cTnI) come close to an ideal marker. Both troponins exist in two pools, one soluble and one structurally bound. Similar to other cytoplasmatic proteins, such as CK, LDH, and myoglobin, this soluble troponin pools may be released rapidly after alterations of plasma membrane permeability, which is at least partly responsible for the early increase in cTnI and cTnT following myocardial damage. The prolonged increase in troponins reflects the dissociation and/or degradation of the contractile apparatus. Soluble

Table 8.1. Characteristics of laboratory parameters for the diagnosis of acute myocardial infarction

Marker	MW (kD)	Biological HLT (h)	Increase (h)	Peak (h) (h)	Normalization (d)
AST (GOT)	93	20	6–12	18–36*	3–4
LDH-1 / HBDH	135	110	6–12	48–144*	7–14
CK	86	17	3–12	12–24*	3–4
CKMB activity	86	13	3–12	12–24*	2–3
CKMB mass	86	13	2–6	12–24*	3
Myoglobin	17.8	0.25	2–6	6–12*	1
MLC-1 and 2	20/26	2–4	4–12	72–120	7–14
MHC	200	?	24–48	96–144	10–14
cTnI	24	2–4	3–8	12–24*	7–10
cTnT	37	2–4	3–8	12–96*	7–14
GPBB	188	4–6	1–4	10–20*	1–2
H-FABP	15	0.3	2–5	6–12*	1

*Strongly dependent on the occurrence of early reperfusion of the infarct-related coronary artery.
Abbreviations: Hours (h), days (d), molecular weight (MW), kiloDalton (kD), half-life time (HLT), aspartate aminotransferase (AST), lactate dehydrogenase (LDH), hydroxybutyrate dehydrogenase (HBDH), creatine kinase (CK), myosin light chains (MLC), myosin heavy chains (MHC), cardiac troponin I (cTnI), cardiac troponin T (cTnT), glycogen phosphorylase BB (GPBB), heart fatty acid-binding protein (H-FABP).

troponin precursor pools and a possible rapid dissociation and degradation of bound troponin allow to monitor the effectiveness of thrombolytic therapy. Early reperfusion causes a more rapid increase in troponins and earlier peaks. The presence of significant soluble troponin precursor pools, however, may also have some disadvantages. There is increasing evidence that cytoplasmatic proteins may be released in small amounts even during the reversible phase of ischemic myocardial injury. Slight troponin increases of short duration, therefore, may not necessarily reflect myocardial necrosis. But prolonged troponin increases for more than 2 days are generally considered to reflect myocardial necrosis. The intracellular compartmentalization of cTnI and cTnT into two pools frequently causes biphasic concentration time courses (particularly for cTnT) after myocardial damage. This hampers the calculation of cumulative troponin release, because more sophisticated mathematical models are necessary than were used for cardiac enzymes. Therefore a marker, such as myosin heavy chains, with a monophasic time course which is not significantly influenced by reperfusion of the infarct-related coronary artery, could be more useful for quantification of myocardial necrosis in absence of concomitant skeletal muscle damage. But this remains to be demonstrated in clinical or experimental studies on the quantification of myocardial infarct size. Because cardiac troponins are not detectable in the reference populations, they are highly specific and sensitive, and more suitable than cardiac enzymes for diagnosing small myocardial damage. This may help to discern the more subtle aspects of myocardial damage, e.g., in cardiotoxicity and myocarditis or the evaluation of cardioprotective measures.

The following recommendations are based on current knowledge (1996), and only already commercially available markers are considered. CKMB mass assays have a higher analytical specificity and a higher diagnostic sensitivity than the currently available CKMB activity assays.[1-5] Despite somewhat higher costs, the recommendation, therefore, is to replace CKMB activity with CKMB mass measurement in the routine laboratory, in particular for CKMB testing in samples which are sent from the emergency department of the hospital. Then, total CK activity measurements are no longer needed in patients with suspected myocardial injury, because CKMB mass determination is at least as sensitive than CK activity measurement. There are no analytical restrictions for the routine use of CKMB mass determination. Rapid assays suitable for emergency determination of CKMB mass and also a semiquantitative whole-blood bedside test are available from various manufacturers. Standardized CKMB mass assays will be available in the near future, which is a prerequisite for the comparison of results obtained with different assays. As long as costs of troponin determination are higher than of CKMB mass measurement cTnI and cTnT should be restricted to patients in whom their high specificity and sensitivity are really required. These are in particular patients with possible concomitant skeletal muscle damage.

ACUTE MYOCARDIAL INFARCTION (AMI)

PATIENTS WITH IMMEDIATE ACUTE PERCUTANEOUS CORONARY ANGIOPLASTY (PTCA)

During recent years immediate angioplasty for AMI has become increasingly popular in cardiological centers experienced in invasive cardiovascular procedures that can perform emergency bypass surgery.[6,7] In particular patients with contraindications to thrombolytic therapy or high risk patients (large anterior infarction, cardiogenic shock or persistent tachycardia) will benefit from this intervention. The decision for immediate coronary angiography is based on ECG findings and the clinical history. Patient management depends on angiographic findings. Biochemical markers are only used for documentation of AMI. Therefore, CKMB measurement according to a usual blood sampling regimen (e.g., every 8-12 hours within the first 24 hours and daily until normalization) is completely sufficient in these patients.

PATIENTS WITH THROMBOLYTIC TREATMENT, MONITORING OF THE EFFECTIVENESS OF THROMBOLYTIC THERAPY

In contrast to immediate PTCA which has limited applicability because of the severely restricted accessibility of the procedure, intravenous thrombolytic therapy is widely available and clearly beneficial in AMI patients. Fibrinolytic therapy is currently advised for patients presenting within 12 hours from chest pain onset (but the earlier therapy is started the more benefits can be expected) and ST segment elevation or presumably new left-bundle branch block in their ECG, regardless of the results of biochemical markers.[8] But the exact relevant time point of chest pain onset is sometimes difficult to define. In this case and if biochemical markers are still not increased and the patient fulfills all the other criteria for administration of thrombolysis, markers may be helpful to decide whether or not to give thrombolytic treatment to patients admitted later than 6-12 hours after chest pain onset.

Unfortunately, there is a 25-30% failure rate of intravenous thrombolytic therapy, and if therapy fails, the patients have a higher risk. Early full patency leads to an improved prognosis over later full patency of the infarct related coronary artery. Coronary angiography is the criterion standard for assessing the patency of the infarct-related coronary artery. But it is an invasive and costly procedure associated with a certain risk in AMI patients. In addition it is not always possible to perform angiography on all patients in most hospitals. Therefore, noninvasive markers were tested to assess reperfusion after starting thrombolysis with the aim to identify those patients who may benefit from early angiography and possibly from rescue angioplasty.

The early rate of increase or relative increase of all cytosolic proteins and of troponins during thrombolytic therapy allow to assess the therapeutic effectiveness with higher diagnostic accuracy than other noninvasive methods (ST monitoring, reperfusion-induced arrythmias, resolution of chest pain).[9,10] The differences of diagnostic performances are small, but myoglobin is tendentiously the best marker,[9] because its diagnostic performance is less susceptible to changes in the threshold value used.[10] If acute coronary angiographies are not routinely performed, it is possible to identify patients with failed reperfusion early by biochemical criteria with acceptable accuracy.[9,10] In many studies reperfusion was defined as thrombolysis in myocardial infarction trial (TIMI) grades 2 or 3 patency (partial or complete reperfusion). In light of recent reports that TIMI grade 3 patency results might indicate positive patient outcome better than TIMI grade 2[11] a more rigorous TIMI 3-only definition of "open" is desirable. This usually decreases the discriminatory power of biochemical markers between "open" and "closed". However, in a recent multicenter study[10] Laperche et al could demonstrate that the differentiation between TIMI 3 grade patients from the others is possible with sufficient accuracy by the relative increase in biochemical markers within 90 minutes from start of thrombolytic therapy. Myoglobin gave tendentiously the best results. However, the results of this study still remain to be tested in a prospective study. There will always be some overlap between the "open" and "closed" groups for several reasons, that are the dynamic nature of patency restoration for many patients, and individual patient variables, such as extent of infarct and collateral flow. In addition angiography assesses patency only for one point in time. Only serial angiographies can discriminate how long it takes to achieve different grades of perfusion in the infarct-related coronary artery.

Thus, it is recommended to combine for the noninvasive assessment of reperfusion the calculation of the early rate of increase or relative increase of a biochemical marker calculated from blood samples drawn before and after stop of thrombolytic therapy with electrocardiographic ST-segment monitoring and clinical indicators.[12]

However, the clinical implications of detecting failed reperfusion are less clear and controversial, which may limit the importance of measurement of biochemical markers for this purpose. Usually the detection of failed reperfusion has no acute clinical consequences. The routine use of rescue PTCA does not appear to offer benefits

beyond that of contemporary medical treatment after thrombolytic
failure, probably because of the high mortality associated with failed
rescue PTCA and the little potential for myocardial salvage at the
time when recue PTCA is performed.[13] However, patients with
cardiogenic shock, pulmonary edema, or a large anterior wall
infarction with persisting signs of myocardial ischemia should have,
whenever possible, emergent cardiac catheterization and rescue
PTCA.[14] However, these patients are usually identified clinically
and intervention is only possible at hospitals with appropriate facilities and operator expertise. In such centers, however, routine
postlytic cardiac catheterization is usually performed, because this
has attractive attributes, including the potential for earlier hospital
discharge.[14]

Blood samples for CKMB mass measurement should be collected in this group of AMI patients according to the common
regimen, that is every 6-8 hours within the first 24 hours and
daily until normalization. If the clinician wants to include biochemical markers for the monitoring of thrombolytic treatment,
additional blood samples before and immediately after stop of
thrombolytic treatment must be drawn to calculate the relative
increase or slope. Currently myoglobin appears to be the most
promising marker for monitoring of thrombolytic therapy.

PATIENTS WITH CONVENTIONAL TREATMENT

Therapeutic decisions do not depend on the results of myocardial marker measurement in these patients. Therefore, blood
samples for CKMB measurement should be collected according to
the usually used regimen, that is every 6-8 hours within the first
24 hours and daily until normalization.

LATE DIAGNOSIS OF MYOCARDIAL INFARCTION

This is not a very frequent problem in daily clinical practice.
For the late diagnosis of AMI in patients presenting later than 1-2
days LDH isoenzyme determination should be replaced by the more
sensitive and specific cTnT or cTnI measurement.

SUSPECTED MYOCARDIAL INFARCTION: EARLY CONFIRMATION OR RULING OUT

The use of an ECG still is the quickest, simplest and most
reliable method for early AMI diagnosis, and in many patients the

diagnosis of AMI is straightforward and not a diagnostic dilemma. Careful assessment of the clinical history and ECG at the time of hospital admission will identify about 80% of all heart attack patients.[15] But there remains an important minority in whom the diagnosis is difficult to establish. In these patients the diagnosis cannot be made with certainty from the ECG and the clinical history, and biochemical markers are a cheap and great help for medical decision making. These patients constitute a group with or without typical infarct-related symptoms that shows ECG patterns which are difficult to interpret because of, e.g., bundle branch block, pace maker or a possible reinfarction. In patients with suspected reinfarction in the region of an old infarction echocardiography also is not very helpful, because it is difficult to decide whether the wall motion abnormalities have recently developed. Similarly difficult is to interpret perfusion myocardial scintigraphies in these patients. Therefore, the increase in myocardial protein markers is the most reliable means of diagnosis. In particular, in smaller hospitals without the possibilities of doing costly coronary angiography, echocardiography or myocardial scintigraphy on a 24 hour basis, laboratory markers are a cornerstone in diagnosing AMI in the difficult cases.

The majority of chest pain patients admitted to the emergency department are sent for ruling out AMI, and only about 10-15% of chest pain patients have AMI. For the exclusion of AMI biochemical markers generally play the more important role. All newer markers (CKMB mass, CK isoforms, myoglobin, cTnI, cTnT) have a roughly equivalent early sensitivity, and the differences are not clinically relevant[3] (see Table 8.2). All are markedly more sensitive than CK and CKMB activity,[3] but during the first 3 hours after the onset of chest pain the diagnostic performance of the ECG is clearly superior to all biochemical markers.[16] However, at hospital presentation the ECG may be nondiagnostic in up to 50% of AMI patients and lacks sensitivity at that time point as well.[4,16] After 3 hours from chest pain onset the discriminatory power of CKMB mass to diagnose AMI defined according to the WHO-criteria was superior to the ECG and the other tested biochemical markers.[16] To exclude an AMI with 100% certainty by negative test results of newer biochemical markers it is still necessary to wait for at least 10 hours from the onset of chest pain.[17] If chest pain reoccurs during this period, it takes even longer.

Table 8.2. Average early sensitivities of commercially available biochemical markers for myocardial damage during the first 6 hours from chest pain onset

Marker	Hours from chest pain onset		
	0 - 2	2 - 4	4 - 6
CK activity	0.15	0.35	0.70
CKMB activity	0.10	0.25	0.50
CKMB mass	0.30	0.70	0.90
CKMM isoform ratio	0.25	0.60	0.85
CKMB isoform ratio	0.25	0.60	0.90
Myoglobin	0.35	0.80	0.95
Cardiac Troponin I	0.30	0.60	0.80
Cardiac Troponin T	0.30	0.55	0.80

In these patients a more close-matched early sampling regimen, e.g., 0, 3, 6, and 9 hours after admission for measurement of either CKMB mass, CK isoforms, or myoglobin, should replace the currently used blood sampling of every 6-8 hours during the first day after admission. This allows to confirm or rule out the diagnosis more quickly and allows to manage patient care accordingly (coronary care unit, monitored bed, general ward, outpatient), which helps to save costs by more efficient use of treatment facilities and expensive coronary care beds. However, it is unclear how earlier diagnosis of AMI with nondiagnostic admission ECG would impact on patient treatment. For patients with nondiagnostic ECG changes (ST segment depression or T wave inversion) thrombolysis should not be given, even when biochemical confirmation of AMI has become available, because it does not confer benefits or may even be harmful.[8,11]

We cannot yet judge what role ward-based marker analysis will eventually have in the early management of heart attack. If it is right to make every effort to get patients into the coronary care unit as quickly as possible after infarction, it must be also right to make an equivalent effort to confirm the diagnosis rapidly. Serial cardiac markers and ST-segment trend monitoring may help to achieve that goal.

DIAGNOSIS OF MYOCARDIAL INFARCTION OR ACUTE MYOCARDIAL INJURY IN PATIENTS WITH CONCOMITANT OR SUSPECTED SKELETAL MUSCLE DAMAGE

Several studies clearly demonstrated that cTnI and cTnT are markedly superior to CK and LDH isoenzymes if AMI has to be diagnosed in patients with possible concomitant skeletal muscle damage, such as in patients after resuscitation, patients with chest pain after heavy physical exercise, or the fainted athlete after competition. For example, the diagnosis of acute myocardial injury in marathon runners is complicated by elevations of CKMB in asymptomatic finishers with normal postrace myocardial scintigraphy, because particularly in endurance-trained athletes CKMB elevations frequently arise from exercise-induced skeletal muscle damage. Only cTnI or cTnT should be measured in these patients. In the great majority of patients the specificities of both troponins are equivalent. cTnI should be preferred in patients with chronic renal failure, multiple organ damage, or chronic myopathies.

NONINVASIVE ESTIMATION OF INFARCT SIZE BY CALCULATION OF CUMULATIVE BIOCHEMICAL MARKER RELEASE

The noninvasive estimation of myocardial infarct size by calculation of the cumulative release of myocardial proteins is one of the most controversial topics in the clinical chemistry of AMI. Estimating infarct size is not a generally accepted indication for measurement of biochemical markers in AMI patients. Imaging techniques are usually superior in the individual patient, because they also provide additional information.

In general, it is desirable that a high percentage of a marker protein is released from the myocardium with little remaining within the infarcted tissue, because this leads to a high precision. Slowly catabolyzed proteins also offer advantages, because errors resulting from the sampling regimen are smaller. The marker should of course be distributed uniformly throughout the myocardium, and coronary artery disease should not alter myocardial marker content.

In reality cumulative marker release can only be transformed to gram equivalents of average healthy tissue. Diseased myocardium has a somewhat lower cardiac enzyme content than healthy tissue. The protein content in the individual patient is of course not known. For the cardiac contractile and regulatory proteins the tissue distribution, release ratios, and effects of diseases on protein content of myocardium are not yet sufficiently investigated. Many researchers have concerns regarding the recovery of proteins from the infarcted tissue. The wash-out from the peripheral zones is usually deemed to be greater than from the central region of the infarct. Therefore, the three-dimensional shape of the infarcted region may influence protein release from the infarcted tissue.

Nonetheless, correlations of cumulative marker release (not necessarily peak values) with other independent methods of quantifying infarct size have been described for all markers also in patients receiving thrombolytic therapy (see respective chapters). However, a superiority of the contractile proteins or troponins over LDH-1 isoenzyme or hydroxybutyrate dehydrogenase (HBDH) to estimate infarct-size has not yet been demonstrated in AMI patients.

PERIOPERATIVE MYOCARDIAL INFARCTION

GENERAL SURGERY

Only cTnI or cTnT should be measured in these patients, because only these two markers allow to definitively diagnose or rule out perioperative myocardial infarction. Daily blood sampling is sufficient. If an earlier detection has therapeutic consequences in the individual patient, blood samples should be collected every 4-6 hours during the first 24 postoperative hours. In the great majority the specificities of both troponins are equivalent. cTnI should be preferred in patients with chronic renal failure, multiple organ damage, or chronic myopathies.

HEART SURGERY—
CORONARY ARTERY BYPASS GRAFTING (CABG)

After CABG the general reference limits are not valid for all cardiac enzymes and proteins as there is inevitable cardiac tissue damage (e.g., by right atriotomy for cannulation, cardioplegic cardiac arrest, or intermittent aortic cross-clamping) occurring during the surgical procedure. Therefore, all markers significantly increase after reperfusion over values seen before bypass also in patients without complications. Myoglobin and other markers which are rapidly cleared from the plasma allow to differentiate between patients with and without perioperative myocardial infarction (PMI) as early as 3 hours after aortic unclamping. cTnI and cTnT appear to be the most sensitive and specific markers to detect minor perioperative myocardial injury in patients who do not fulfill the standard PMI criteria. Perioperative myocardial cell damage seems to be much more common than has been previously recognized by changes of ECG and serum enzyme activities.

The clinical implications of measuring these new markers in CABG patients are not fully delineated so far. It remains to be clearly demonstrated that the earlier detection of PMI by myoglobin measurement has a significant influence on patient care. But without doubt knowing that the patient has developed a PMI, for example, facilitates the decision to use intraaortic balloon pumping for circulatory support. In addition, the clinical and prognostic significance of detecting minor perioperative myocardial damage in CABG patients remains to be demonstrated in a large prospective multicenter trial.

In summary, the laboratory is now able to offer cardiac surgeons and cardiovascular anesthesiologists a panel of new markers which allow to rapidly discriminate between patients with and without PMI and to detect minor myocardial injury in CABG patients. cTnI and cTnT may be very useful for quality control in CABG patients, e.g., by assessing the effectiveness of various cardioprotective measures. Daily blood sampling for cTnI or cTnT measurement until the 4th postoperative day is sufficient.

Separate postsurgical discriminator values of biochemical markers have to be evaluated for other cardiac surgical procedures, especially if they include cardiotomy, e.g., mitral valve surgery and CABG during the same operation. For all other cardiac surgical procedures (e.g., valve replacements in patients without coronary artery disease, corrections of malformations of the heart) PMI is fortunately a rare complication. If surgical procedures include cardiotomy with surgical trauma to the heart also cTnI and cTnT are not very helpful markers in these patients.

RISK STRATIFICATION IN PATIENTS WITH UNSTABLE ANGINA PECTORIS

The decision with which emergency physicians in chest pain patients are confronted is not just to simply rule in or rule out AMIs, it is more important to discriminate chest pain patients with no or stable coronary artery disease from those with acute coronary syndromes. Acute coronary syndromes encompass the entities AMI, unstable angina pectoris, and sudden ischemic death. They are caused by an active coronary plaque, the culprit lesion. This is often the site of intermittent occlusion and of thrombotic formation with episodic microembolization, with or without vasospasm. 5-20% of patients with unstable angina have a poor prognosis with progression to AMI or cardiac death within the first year. Even if AMI could be ruled out in chest pain patients, it is important to identify high risk patients with unstable angina early to prevent the progression of the disease to AMI or cardiac death.

Biochemical markers are useful for early risk stratification in chest pain patients. By serial sampling in patients with unstable angina Ravkilde et al found that the prognostic value of CKMB mass, myosin light chains, and cTnT is equivalent.[2] In this study marker protein increase, however, could not add additional prognostic information to ECG, that is ECG signs for myocardial ischemia at rest.[2] However, recent data on risk stratification in patients with acute coronary syndromes of the GUSTO-IIa and FRISC trials[18,19] demonstrated that cTnT is an independent risk factor (higher values are associated with increasing rates of cardiac events) and that cTnT concentrations were significantly more strongly associated with mortality than CKMB mass concentrations. The admission cTnT concentration provided the most important risk stratification. Comparable large studies on the prognostic significance of cTnI increase in patients with unstable angina are not yet available, but first results on cTnI are promising and it is very likely that cTnI is comparable with the other already tested markers. Troponins are somewhat more frequently increased in patients with unstable angina than CKMB mass concentrations. Of patients with increased myocardial markers 20-40% suffer cardiac death or AMI within the subsequent months, compared to only 5-10% if biochemical markers are not increased.

As the ECG is frequently difficult to interpret in unstable angina and cTnT is an independent risk factor, an early risk stratification based on clinical history, ECG,[20,21] and myocardial markers is recommended. Measurement of markers on admission, 12 and 24 hours later is sufficient. Current studies try to prove the cost-effectiveness of troponin measurements in patients with acute coronary syndromes. The hypothesis to prove is that therapeutic interventions (coronary angiography and revascularization procedures) in patients with increases in troponin improve their prognosis by preventing a major cardiac event.

MARKER PROTEIN RELEASE AFTER INVASIVE CARDIOLOGICAL PROCEDURES

After PTCA or other invasive cardiological procedures, sensitive biochemical markers, such as cTnI, cTnT, and CKMB mass or CK isoforms, are more frequently increased over baseline values than cardiac enzyme activities. However, the clinical and prognostic implications of detecting this limited myocardial injury are not sufficiently investigated and known so far. The clinical impact has to be clearly demonstrated before it is justified to include the measurement of these markers as part of the routine evaluation of patients undergoing invasive cardiological procedures. However, these sensitive markers are important for quality control and comparison of different methods and may be an important endpoint of clinical trials.

NONISCHEMIC MYOCARDIAL DAMAGE

MYOCARDITIS

Experimental and first clinical results clearly indicate that cTnI and cTnT are more sensitive markers for this disease than CKMB. Therefore, cTnI or cTnT should replace CKMB determination in patients with suspected myocarditis. Elevations in patients with clinically suspected myocarditis indicate the disease, but negative results do not exclude its presence. In cases with mainly interstitial inflammatory infiltrates myocyte necrosis is not prominent and marker elevations may be absent. A comparative study on the diagnostic performances of cTnI and cTnT in patients with suspected myocarditis has not been performed so far (1996). Increases in troponins are prolonged in patients with acute myocarditis. Frequently there is no pronounced peak value. Daily blood sampling for troponin measurement is sufficient.

HEART CONTUSION

One of the most feared complications of chest trauma is myocardial contusion. However, the extent of investigation and management of less symptomatic, hemodynamically stable patients remains controversial. For the laboratory diagnosis of heart contusion CKMB should be replaced by cTnI or cTnT measurement. The use of tests as predictors for complications is, however, more useful than establishing the diagnosis.[22] CKMB determinations are not very helpful for estimating prognosis in patients with heart contu-

---

Table 8.3. Summary

Disease
    Interpretation

Myocardial infarction (early diagnosis)
    Semiquantitative whole blood bedside assays for the rapid determination of myoglobin, CKMB mass, troponin T and troponin I are easy to perform and to interpret. However, the results of a single measurement must be assessed with caution. Within the first 6 hours from chest pain onset only the positive result is a real help for clinical decision making. For ruling out a suspected myocardial infarction with certainty, one has to wait for the test result after 10 hours from chest pain onset. This time period is longer, if significant chest pain reoccurs during the observation period.

Myocardial infarction (late diagnosis)
    In patients presenting 1-2 days after the onset of acute infarct-related symptoms the determination of LDH isoenzymes for the laboratory diagnosis of infarction will be replaced by the more sensitive and specific markers cardiac troponin I and troponin T.

Monitoring of thrombolytic therapy in patients with acute myocardial infarction
    In principal the monitoring is possible by calculation of the rate of increase or relative increase of every cytosolic marker or troponin T and troponin I. Reperfusion leads to a more rapid increase in these markers and peak values occur earlier. If concomitant skeletal muscle damage can be excluded clinically, myoglobin was found to be tendentiously the best marker to discriminate between patients with and without early reperfusion. A relative increase in myoglobin >4 within 90 minutes after start of thrombolytic treatment indicates successful reperfusion (TIMI grade III, complete reperfusion) with high accuracy.

Tachycardia, heart failure, valvular heart disease
    Usually myocardial proteins are not increased in these patients. In a subgroup of patients with cardiomyopathies increases in CK isoforms, CKMB mass, and cardiac troponins were described. This is probably explained by disease progression with ongoing myocardial damage.

Perioperative myocardial infarction, heart contusion, myocarditis
    Due to their higher specificity cardiac troponin I and troponin T are the markers of choice for diagnosing myocardial damage in presence of concomitant skeletal muscle injury. In patients with myocarditis also troponins are not 100% sensitive (increases are rarely seen in patients with focal, primarily interstitial infiltrates).

sions, and future studies on troponins in heart contusion should
focus on this issue rather than just trying to prove their usefulness
for diagnostic purposes.

The overall prognosis of the stable chest trauma is excellent
and complete recovery is the rule.[22] Patients can be discharged from
the hospital after 24 hours of monitoring their ECG and troponin

---

Table 8.3. Summary (continued)

Disease
   Interpretation

Coronary artery bypass grafting
   Due to the inevitable myocardial damage from cannulation (usually includes
   right atriotomy), cardioplegic cardiac arrest, or intermittent aortic crossclamping
   all myocardial proteins increase even in uncomplicated patients. Therefore,
   only increases in CKMB mass >50 µg/L, and troponin T or troponin I >2.5 µg/
   L 12-20 hours after aortic unclamping indicate perioperative myocardial
   infarction.

**Myocardial damage in patients with severe renal failure, multiple organ
damage, or patients with chronic myopathy**
   According to current knowledge cardiac troponin I should be used to
   diagnose myocardial damage in these patients.

Stable angina pectoris
   Myocardial protein markers are not increased in patients with stable angina.

**Unstable angina pectoris, risk stratification in patients with acute coronary
syndromes**
   Myocardial markers (e.g. troponin T, troponin I, CKMB mass) are increased in
   a subgroup of patients with unstable angina pectoris. Patients with increase in
   markers have a worse prognosis (similar to that of AMI patients) than patients
   without increases. Additional diagnostic cardiological examinations (e.g.
   coronary angiography) and interventions are necessary in these patients to
   prevent cardiac events. Currently most data on risk stratification are available
   using troponin T, and this marker is therefore at present the marker of choice
   in these patients.

Diagnostic and invasive-interventional therapeutic cardiological procedures
   Exercise stress tests with or without invasive hemodynamic monitoring,
   coronary angiographies, and uncomplicated coronary angioplasty do not lead
   to an increase in serum concentrations of myocardial marker proteins. After
   myocardial biopsies, resuscitation, direct-current countershock therapy also
   heart-specific markers may be slightly increased. After radiofrequency ablation
   therapy, coronary stent implantation, directional coronary atherectomy and
   related procedures (e.g. coronary rotational ablation) slightly increased marker
   concentrations may be found even in clinically uncomplicated patients.

levels, if results are negative and no other major injuries are present. Troponins should be measured every 8-12 hours during the first 24 hours after admission. It is reasonable to reserve imaging studies for patients with an abnormal ECG and/or troponin level or preexisting cardiac disease.

REJECTION OF THE TRANSPLANTED HEART

After orthotopic heart transplantation all myocardial markers moderately increase. CKMB and CKMB isoform ratio usually normalize within a few days. In contrast to CKMB and CKMB isoform ratio, troponins remain detectable in these patients for up to 4 weeks (cTnI) and 2-3 months (cTnT) even without episodes of acute rejection. This behavior of troponins makes the markers less useful for the detection of episodes of rejection than markers which more rapidly normalize after heart transplantation, because frequent blood sampling is necessary to recognize new increases. Therefore, CKMB mass or CKMB isoforms should be used as laboratory markers of myocardial damage within the first month from transplantation. Thereafter, cTnI may be preferred because of its cardiacspecificity. A principal limitation of all intramyocardial proteins when used for the early detection of rejection episodes is that they only increase when myocardial damage has already occurred. Consequently, a combination of markers of immunoactivation with myocardial proteins may be more suitable for the monitoring of heart transplanted patients. This may be helpful for the differentiation of infections from acute episodes of rejection. An appropriate combination with a suitable blood sampling regimen has to be evaluated in a prospective trial. It remains to be seen whether these laboratory markers can help to reduce the frequency of necessary routine endomyocardial biopsies for the monitoring of possible rejection episodes in patients after heart transplantation.

cTnT and cTnI can be also used to assess the heart in a potential heart transplant donor. The quality of the donor's heart is an important prognostic factor in heart transplantation. In contrast to CKMB, donor cTnT and cTnI are useful predictors of early allograft dysfunction and may influence the decision to use the heart for transplantation.

DIAGNOSIS OF MYOCARDIAL INJURY IN COMPLEX CLINICAL SETTINGS

SEVERE RENAL FAILURE OR MULTIPLE ORGAN FAILURE

In these patients cTnI should be used to diagnose or exclude myocardial injury.

PATIENTS WITH CHRONIC MYOPATHIES

As long as the issue of a possible reexpression of cTnT in the skeletal muscles of patients with chronic muscle diseases has not been fully delineated, cTnI should be used for diagnosis of myocardial injury to be on the safe side.

REFERENCES

1. Mair J, Artner-Dworzak E, Dienstl A et al. Early detection of acute myocardial infarction by measurement of mass concentration of creatine kinase-MB. Am J Cardiol 1991; 68:1545-50.
2. Ravkilde J, Nissen H, Horder M et al. Independent prognostic value of serum creatine kinase isoenzyme MB mass, cardiac troponin T and myosin light chain levels in suspected myocardial infarction. J Am Coll Cardiol 1995; 25:574-81.
3. Mair J, Morandell D, Genser N et al. Equivalent early sensitivities of myoglobin, creatine kinase MB mass, creatine kinase isoform ratios, and cardiac troponin I and T for acute myocardial infarction. Clin Chem 1995; 41:1266-72.
4. Gibler WB, Lewis LM, Erb RE et al. Early detection of acute myocardial infarction in patients presenting with nondiagnostic ECGs: serial CK-MB sampling in the emergency department. Ann Emerg Med 1990; 19:1359-66.
5. Chan KM, Ladenson JH, Pierce GF et al. Increased creatine kinase MB in the absence of acute myocardial infarction. Clin Chem 1986; 32:2044-51.
6. Lange RA, Hillis DL. Immediate angioplasty for acute myocardial infarction. New Engl J Med 1993; 328:726-8.
7. Stewart RE, O'Neill WW. Direct angioplasty for acute myocardial infarction. Curr Opin Cardiol 1995; 10:367-71.
8. Madias JE. Acute myocardial infarction: shifting paradigms of diagnosis and care in cost-conscious environment. Chest 1995; 108:1483-5.
9. Zabel M, Hohnloser SH, Köster W et al. Analysis of creatine kinase, CK-MB, myoglobin, and troponin T time-activity curves for early assessment of coronary artery reperfusion after intravenous thrombolysis. Circulation 1993; 87:1542-50.

10. Laperche T, Steg PG, Dehoux M et al. A study of biochemical markers of reperfusion early after thrombolysis for acute myocardial infarction. Circulation 1995; 92:2079-86.
11. Grover A, Rihal CS. The importance of early patency after acute myocardial infarction. Curr Opin Cardiol 1995; 10:361-6.
12. Doevendans PA, Gorgels AP, van der Zee R et al. Electrocardiographic diagnosis of reperfusion during thrombolytic therapy in acute myocardial infarction. Am J Cardiol 1995; 75:1206-10.
13. McKendall GR, Forman S, Sopko G et al. Value of rescue percutaneous transluminal coronary angioplasty following unsuccessful thrombolytic therapy in patients with acute myocardial infarction. Am J Cardiol 1995; 76:1108-11.
14. Aguirre FV, Merritt RF, Carollo SC. The role of coronary angiography after thrombolysis. Curr Opin Cardiol 1995; 10:381-8.
15. Rude RE, Poole WK, Muller JE et al. Electrocardiographic and clinical criteria for recognition of acute myocardial infarction based on analysis of 3697 patients. Am J Cardiol 1983; 52:936-42.
16. Mair J, Smidt J, Lechleitner P et al. A decision tree for the early diagnosis of acute myocardial infarction in non-traumatic chest pain patients at hospital admission. Chest 1995; 108:1502-9.
17. Bakker AJ, Koelemay MJW, Gorgels JPMC et al. Failure of new biochemical markers to exclude acute myocardial infarction at admission. Lancet 1993; 342:1220-2.
18. Ohman EM, Armstrong P, Califf RM, O'Hanesian MA, Hamm CW, Katus HA, Granger CB, Christenson RH, Cianciolo C, Topol EJ. Risk stratification in acute ischaemic syndromes using serum troponin T. J Am Coll Cardiol1995; 25:148A.
19. Lindahl B, Toss H, Venge P, Wallentin L. Troponin T is an independent prognostic marker for subsequent cardiac events in patients with unstable coronary artery disease (abstract). Circulation 1995; 92 (Suppl 1): 3182.
20. Betriu A, Heras M, Cohen M et al. Unstable angina: outcome according to clinical presentation. J Am Coll Cardiol 1992; 19:1659-63.
21. Rizik DG, Healy S, Margulis A et al. A new clinical classification for hospital prognosis of unstable angina pectoris. Am J Cardiol 1995; 75:993-7.
22. Feghali NT, Prisant ML. Blunt cardiac injury. Chest 1995; 108:1673-7.

CHAPTER 9

CONCLUSION

Currently there is a tendency, in particular in the USA, to try to confirm or exclude the diagnosis of an acute myocardial infarction (AMI) within a few hours, and even to fully evaluate the patient without AMI before discharge, all within 24 hours and in the emergency department to save costs. The chest pain diagnostic and treatment centers have emerged as divisions of the emergency department.[1] Using new myocardial markers (e.g., CKMB mass, CK isoforms, myoglobin, troponins) once after admission, and serially at short time intervals has become increasingly popular as a part of a strategy to rapidly rule out AMI in chest pain patients. This has been recognized by assay manufacturers who compete for this currently booming market. Indeed serial measurement of highly sensitive early markers for rapidly ruling out AMI may be one major application of new laboratory markers for myocardial injury. Because the differences in early sensitivities of different markers are small and hardly of clinical relevance, the choice of a marker should be mainly based on practicability of methods, specificity, and costs. Another important application of new markers is early risk stratification in patients with unstable angina, and for this purpose cardiac troponin T (cTnT) and troponin I (cTnI) are the most promising markers. There is no doubt that the availability of highly sensitive and specific assays for measurement of cTnI and cTnT is a breakthrough for the laboratory diagnosis of myocardial injury in presence of concomitant skeletal muscle damage. Current results suggest that in patients with severe chronic renal functional impairment, multiple organ damage, or chronic myopathies cTnI is the most heart-specific marker.

As costs for troponin measurement decrease, CKMB will be gradually replaced by troponin measurement in all patients with suspected myocardial injury. If it can be definitively demonstrated that human skeletal muscle may reexpress cTnT in clinical settings where cTnI is not expressed, cTnI will become the new criterion standard for the laboratory diagnosis of myocardial damage. In this case and if the first very promising clinical results on glycogen phosphorylase BB (GPBB) can be confirmed in larger groups of patients, the future scenario for the laboratory testing for myocardial injury could be the combination of cTnI and GPBB measurement which combines absolute cardiac specificity with high early sensitivity for ischemic myocardial damage.

In summary, the laboratory is now able to offer clinicians a panel of new markers which are clearly superior to the conventional CKMB and CK activity measurements. They allow, e.g., to detect AMIs earlier and small myocardial damage more accurately even in presence of concomitant skeletal muscle damage. These markers may have a strong impact on patient care. However, in many clinical settings the clinical relevance of measurement of these new biochemical markers still remains to be clearly demonstrated. Additional large multicenter studies are required and are partly already initiated to prove the clinically relevance and cost effectiveness of measuring new laboratory parameters of myocardial injury for patient management and estimation of prognosis in patients.

REFERENCES

1. Graff L, Joseph T, Andelman R et al. American college of emergency physicians information paper: chest pain units in emergency departments—a report from the short-term observation services section. Am J Cardiol 1995; 76:1036-9.

INDEX

A
actin, 74, 79
adenosine diphosphate (ADP), 35, 170
adenosine monophophate (AMP), 122, 171-172
adenosine triphosphate (ATP), 34-36, 38, 77-78, 162,
    166, 170-172
Anderson PAW, 81
arrhythmias, 19-20
aspartate aminotransferase (AST), 1, 13, 27-28
    c-AST, 27-28
    m-AST, 27-28

B
Bachmaier K, 94
Bodor G, 82

C
carbonic anhydrase isoenzyme III, 140-142
cardiomyopathies, 19
chromatofocusing chromatography, 58-59
CKBB (CK-1), 35-36, 38-40, 49
    CKMB (CK-2), 2, 13,18-20, 33-34, 36-39, 69, 80,
        82, 88, 95, 98, 106-111, 121, 127-128, 135,
        144-145, 178, 186, 191, 196, 198, 202
        activity, 17, 72, 84, 94, 165
        clinical significance of, 42-43
        determination, 68, 115
        elimination of, 38
        isoenzyme, 1, 59-60, 73
        mass, 40, 56, 86, 92, 118, 124, 126, 132, 185,
            188-190, 194-195
        pitfalls of, 41
        protein concentration of, 49-56
        release, 113
    CKMB/CK ratio, 14, 20, 41, 140, 142
    CKMM (CK-3), 35-37, 39-40, 49, 56-57, 59, 62-63,
        65-66
        coronary artery bypass grafting (CABG), 15, 54-56,
            63, 71, 89-91, 104-105, 113, 117, 126-127,
            135-137, 192-193
coronary rotational ablation, 102-103
Coxackie B, 19
creatine, 162-166
creatine kinase (CK), 34, 113, *122f*, 123, 127,
        173-174, 177, 179, 183
    activity, 1, 57, 165, 185
    elimination of, 38
    isoenzymes, 39, 49
    isoforms, 56-66, 118, 190, 195
    role of, in muscle metabolism, 34-35
    tissue distribution of, 36-38
creatine phosphate (CP), 34, 163
    levels, 36
Cummins B, 98

D
directional coronary atherectomy (DCA), 102-103
Duchenne muscular dystrophy, 82

E
echocardiography, 12, 15, 20
    electrocardiography (ECG), 1, 6, 8-11, 14-15,
        17-18, 50, 55, 68, 90, 92, 105, 109, 118, 171,
        186, 188-190, 193-194, 197-198
    abnormalities, 19
electrophoresis, 57
enolase isoenzyme $\alpha\beta$, 144

G
glycogen phosphorylase (GP), 119, *122f*, 173
    GPBB, 118-128, 123-127, 202
        clinical use of, 127-128
        diagnostic specificity of, 127
    GPLL, 119, 121
    GPMM, 119, 121
Gotsman MS, 6

H
heart fatty acid binding protein (H-FABP), 128-140
high performance capillary electrophoresis (HPCE), 59
high pressure liquid chromatography (HPLC), 59, 166
2-hydroxybutyrate dehyrogenase (HBDH), 32-33,
    131, 135

I
isoelectric focusing, 58

J
Jennings RB, 6

K
Karmen A, 1
Katus HA, 81, 91, 97
Kobayashi S, 96

L
lactate, 161-162
    lactate dehydrogenase (LDH), 1, 13, 16-17, 28-33,
        43, 47, 74, 82, 107, 113, 130-131, 174, 179,
        183, 188, 191
    LDH-1, 14, 19, 29-33, 88, 111, 113, 115, 121,
        179, 192
    LDH-2, 29-32
    LDH-3, 30-31
    LDH-4, 30-31
    LDH-5, 29-32
Ladue JS, 1